# REFLECTIONS OF A FORTUNATE FELLOW

# Reflections of a Fortunate Fellow

*by*

Professor Geoffrey L. Howe

The Memoir Club

First published in 2002 by
The Memoir Club
Whitworth Hall
Spennymoor
County Durham



British Library Cataloguing in
Publication Data.
A catalogue record for this book
is available from the
British Library.

ISBN: 1 84104 023 1

Typeset by George Wishart & Associates, Whitley Bay.
Printed by Bookcraft (Bath) Ltd.

*In memory of my wonderful and*
*inspiring wife and our treasured only son.*

# Contents

# List of Illustrations

# Foreword
## by Professor Sir Paul Bramley

IN A BAR IN ZURICH three young men sat around enjoying a drink. The conversation turned to life ambition. Geoffrey Howe said he wanted to make a real contribution to better the future of his profession. We did not comment.

I had no idea that 40 years later I would be writing a foreword to this book which describes the fulfilment of that dream.

It is a frank account of a remarkably busy and eventful life of service and I am amazed at his powers of recall for names and places: but then he is an exceptional man. Being a strong person blessed with abundant energy, brains and drive, he inevitably has collected at each stage in life much friendship, appreciation and even adulation. But at the same time he has acquired uncomfortable enemies.

Konrad Lorenz described experiments with the living space of rats. As the cages became progressively smaller so the aggressive behaviour of the rats increased. There seems to be some human parallel of these experiments judging by Professor Howe's experiences in enclosed institutions such as at Newcastle, the Royal Dental Hospital, the Prince Philip Hospital, Hong Kong and in Jordan.

His contemporaries will find the descriptions of his earlier life evocative of a much tougher social scene than we know today. Such retrospection certainly gives us a more healthy appreciation of those who brought us up and gave us our first opportunities. Opportunities Geoffrey has had in abundance and has said 'yes' to them, often at personal risk and he has delivered. 'It is a wise man who makes his own good fortune.'

Flexibility is one of the hallmarks of a top-grade person. This book demonstrates his diverse contributions in clinical service, teaching, publication, research and the national and international politics of his profession. He also clearly relished and made time for a life outside of work.

Colleagues in the dental and medical professions will read this work avidly and have pleasure in identifying with so many events and happenings he describes. Perhaps they will also have the unworthy ambition of wanting to see if their names are mentioned or maybe relieved if they are not mentioned. They will also want to know whether they are on his black list!

The general reader will see, in this story of one man's life, a microcosm of the joys, frustrations, sheer hard work and dedication of a professional life.

## Chapter One

# Early Days

FOR REASONS WHICH, I trust, will soon become obvious to the reader, my memories of childhood are fragmentary and my knowledge of my forbears is largely anecdotal.

I can only recall meeting my father's mother once or twice. She was a talented and good looking professional singer who, after being left a young widow with a baby daughter, married my paternal grandfather, a young widower with one son. He was, by trade, a craftsman joiner and was stone deaf for most of his life. Unfortunately, by the time that I arrived on the scene he had also become blind, making communication between us difficult to say the least.

They had a large family of which my father, Leo Leslie John Howe, was the youngest but one. Like many other theatrical folk my grandmother had a heart of gold and gave a home to two or three waifs one of whom, my 'Uncle' John, was Chinese. In 1914 my father's stepbrother had the doubtful distinction of being one of the first, if not the very first, British soldier to die on British soil of wounds sustained in France, when he expired whilst being transferred from ship to shore in Dover. Perhaps because of this event my father, who was fifteen years of age at the time, ran away from home, lied about his age and joined the York and Lancaster Regiment. He served in Italy and took part in the disastrous Battle of Caparetto when our Italian allies were routed by the Austrians. His true age was then discovered and he was taken out of the front line for the rest of the war. After being demobilised he was employed by Pathè, one of the earliest pioneer filmmakers, to promote and distribute their products and met my mother whilst both were queuing to enter a music hall.

My maternal grandmother was of Huguenot descent, as portrayed by her maiden name, Boutel. She grew up in Lavenham and Long Melford, Suffolk and was the daughter of one of the first engine drivers on the Great Eastern Railway. This must have been comparable with being a Concorde pilot today. It certainly paid well for he lived in some style in a large mansion standing it its own grounds, with his wife and fourteen children, only one of whom was a boy. None of the girls was either educated or expected to go out to work. They were brought up to be ladies and all but one of them married. Soon after giving my grandmother away at her wedding in Ely Cathedral he was killed in a bizarre railway accident whilst driving a train engine in thick fog. He leaned out of his cab looking for the signal on which he struck his head.

When my grandmother was about eleven years old she was found to be anaemic and was instructed by the family doctor to drink a Guinness a day. This prescription was faithfully honoured until she died in her late eighties. She always referred to the beverage as her medicine and grimaced as she drank it. Her husband, my grandfather, was a classical Victorian father and very much the head of the family who sported a large moustache which he waxed assiduously. He was an engineer who specialised in building and ventilating bank vaults, and was extremely conservative in outlook and positive in his beliefs. A good husband and father, no doubt, but being a bit of a martinet, hardly the easiest person to live with. He was passionate about his prize geraniums and spent his leisure hours tending them with his pipe firmly clenched between his teeth and his greenhouse full of tobacco smoke. It was immediately apparent to anyone who came within range of him, at any time, that he was an extremely heavy smoker!

In later life he developed arthritis in his knees and used to attend the Physiotherapy Clinic two or three times each week, wearing the longest pair of short trousers that I have ever seen. I well remember the day that he was told there was nothing more that they could do for him. My grandmother and I were sitting in the lounge when we heard his key in the front door. Using his walking stick in a very noisy fashion he slowly progressed down the passage, flung the lounge door open and waving his stick in the air, announced that he was crippled for life! As he was more than eighty years old at the time and I was still in my teens I found this performance amusing and so incurred his displeasure.

My mother, Ada Blanche Partridge, was the youngest of his three children and my uncle, Sidney Herbert Partridge, of whom I write later, was the eldest and the apple of his father's eye. The family lived first in Holloway, close to his employer's premises and later in Harringay in North London. My mother was extremely bright and industrious and, unusually for a girl in those days, won a scholarship to grammar school where she excelled in her studies. Despite this fact and the urgent pleas of her teachers my grandfather made her leave school when she was fifteen years of age and become a Trainee Sales Assistant at Messrs Bourne and Hollingsworth, the West End department store. She later obtained employment as a clerk in the Bank of England.

In the meantime, my Uncle Sid, a pre war soldier in the Territorial Army (Middlesex Regiment), was mobilised in 1914 and served in Mesopotamia, France and Belgium. After one battle in which he was one of only four survivors in his battalion, a blessing that he always attributed to his small stature, he was transferred to the London Rifle Brigade of which he was a staunch supporter for the rest of his long life. In 1916 a mortar bomb landed in his outpost killing a number of his colleagues and wounding the rest. He lost half of one foot and sustained multiple and severe leg injuries. According to him the German troops who overran the outpost were very young and were bayoneting all the wounded who could not walk, when a Captain in the Queen Victoria Rifles, who had two broken arms, picked him up and carried him over his shoulder for two miles into captivity. My uncle again attributed his survival to his small stature and on his return to the UK moved heaven and earth to ensure that the officer's gallantry was recognised, until it was by the award of the Distinguished Service Order.

Back in England he had been reported as being 'Missing believed killed' and all his family, especially his father, were distraught. About this time my mother had fallen in love with a senior colleague in the Bank of England who, despite being called Mr English, was in fact a Swiss national of German descent. She made the mistake of bringing him home to meet her family, for on hearing his Germanic accent my grandfather flew into a rage, threw him down the steps and severely restricted her leisure activities, a prelude to later events.

My uncle finished up in a hospital near Leipzig and in common with his captors endured many privations, even being so hungry as to eat rat soup. He was not well enough to be repatriated until almost a year after the Armistice was signed, but just about survived the long journey across Europe by train, ship and motor ambulance. On arrival at a British military hospital his condition was described as being 'very poorly' and amputation of his leg was advised as being essential to improve his chances of survival. However my grandparents adamantly refused to agree to this and he was condemned to a lengthy and incomplete recovery before his rehabilitation could begin. It was decided that he would have to earn his living whilst sitting down and so he was offered training as either a watchmaker/jeweller or a dental technician. He chose the latter and was sent to work in the dental laboratory of a private practice in Holloway.

In those days the Royal College of Surgeons of England used to grant exemption from the laboratory year of the Dental Surgery course to those candidates who had spent two years working in a recognised dental laboratory. The establishment to which my uncle was sent happened to be one such facility recognised by the Royal College for this purpose and so he found himself surrounded by able bodied potential dental students. He became extremely popular with them and acquired the nickname 'Birdy' Partridge which he kept for the rest of his long life. He lived to attain the ripe old age of ninety-two and a bit years, and had an important influence on my life at a critical time, as will emerge. It was my pleasure to acknowledge this when I was privileged to give the eulogy at his funeral.

But back to my story. Being a determined and courageous person he overcame many difficulties to learn to stand and walk again, albeit in specially made boots. He was never again to be able to wear shoes. By the time he had achieved this, his new found friends had entered Dental School and

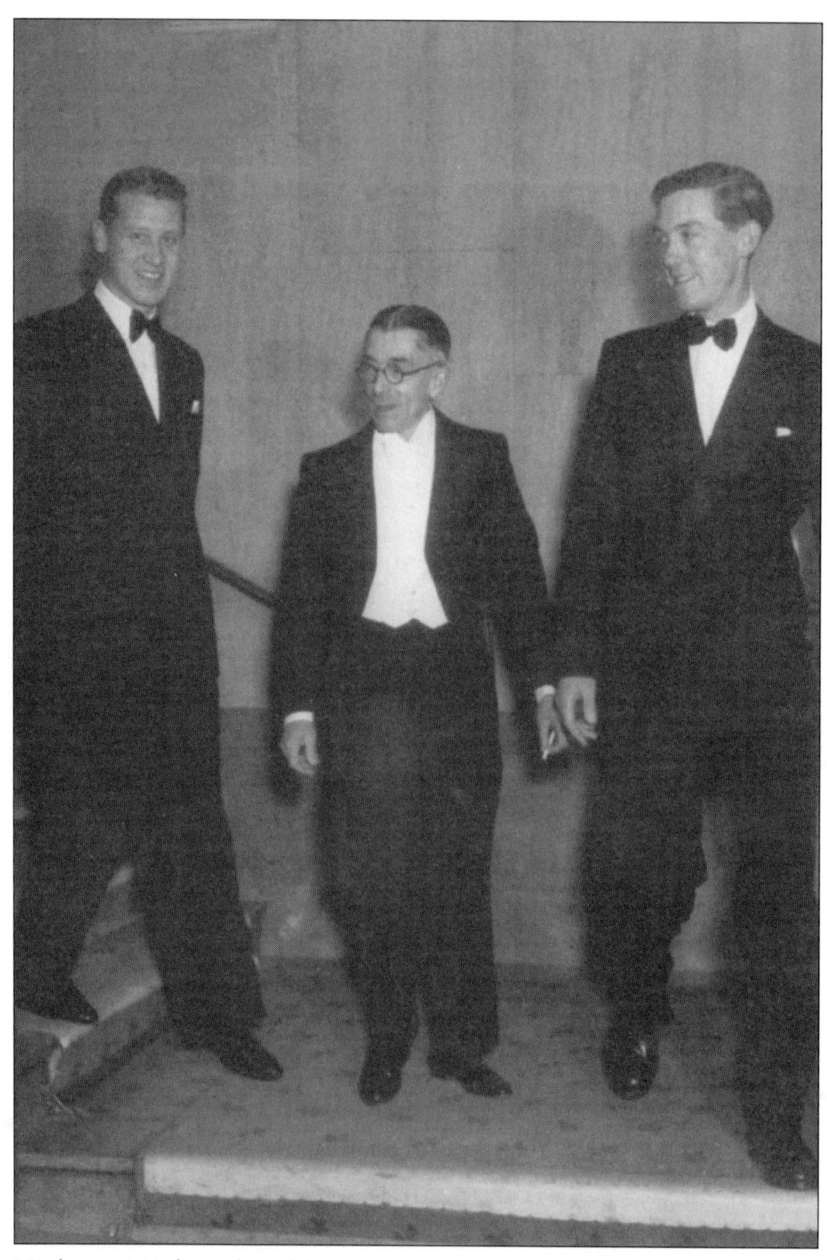

*With my Uncle Sid and brother Alan at the Centenary Dinner of the Royal Dental Hospital and School, 1958.*

were urging him to join them there. After discussions with the pension authorities and with the support of my grandfather, and his life savings, he entered the Royal Dental Hospital of London School of Dental Surgery in Leicester Square, later to be my Alma Mater and that of my younger brother, Alan; but more of that later. He had a distinguished academic record, and made up for his inability to play ball games by actively participating in social activities and student escapades, and qualified with the LDS RCS(Eng) diploma in 1924, the year of my birth. He went on to build up a very successful and ethical general practice from scratch in the Green Lanes, Harringay. Like his father, his standards were extremely high and he was an exacting taskmaster as I soon learned when I became one of his assistants in the practice many years later. He was an adornment to his profession of which he was inordinately proud.

In the post First World War period my father and mother had met, fallen in love, and decided to get married. However, her family were adamantly opposed to their union and created many obstacles to her achieving her desire. Nevertheless, having inherited the family stubbornness and strength of character, she went ahead and married my father, against their wishes, and so became estranged from them. This situation was largely responsible for our relative isolation for almost all of my childhood from the folk described previously; the other factor being poverty. I knew little or nothing about any of them until my mid teens.

I was the eldest of three brothers, and my father died when I was ten years old. I never knew him to be fit and well for unfortunately he had acquired pulmonary tuberculosis, perhaps in the trenches, before I was born. His efforts to build a future for himself and his family were constantly interrupted by sojourns in TB sanatoria, each of which lasted between three and six months. As at that time there was no active treatment for this accursed and widespread killer disease every time he went into hospital he lost his job and when he came out he found it increasingly difficult to find work, for these were times of industrial unrest and the Great Depression was developing. Furthermore, tuberculosis was a dreaded disease, and those afflicted with it, and their families, were treated like lepers by many folk, including some employers. I believe that he worked for a firm called Paton Calvert who made pressed metallic products and the Thames Valley Traction Company as a bus driver, amongst others. We lived in a series of locations around the then borders of Berkshire and Buckinghamshire, in places such as Stoke Poges, Cox's Green, Desborough Park and Clare Road, Maidenhead where we were when he died. He quite literally was prepared to do any job, however menial, to provide for us. However, he put his periods of enforced inactivity to good use for he realised that having left school early in order to volunteer for the Army, he had much to learn. He developed considerable skills in bookkeeping and wrote in a beautiful copperplate script. He borrowed many books on such subjects as theology, philosophy and sociology from the Carnegie Public Libraries and read them assiduously.

He became a Quaker convert and was deeply involved in their various schemes designed to alleviate some of the miseries of unemployment. The Society of Friends believed that it was important to preserve the dignity and morale of the unemployed by encouraging and enabling them to help themselves, rather than relying on either handouts or others.

To this end they provided the able bodied unemployed with allotments, gardening tools and seeds at a nominal charge and encouraged them to grow food to feed their families. Any produce that was surplus to their own needs was bought from them and distributed to those who were either too old, infirm or incapacitated to actively participate in the scheme. My father implemented these activities in the South of England and also arranged for food waste to be regularly collected from hotels and restaurants and fed to pigs by the unemployed, which provided them with meat. It was necessary for him to travel extensively in order to oversee the implementation of both the allotment and pig swill schemes and to resolve problems when and where they arose. He did this in an ancient Austin 7 car and from the age of eight often took me with him on these trips, having taught me what to do if he was taken ill for he knew that his health was failing. The Quakers next sent some fishing boats, which had been laid up, out to sea and arranged for the fish that they caught to be transported and sold cheaply to the unemployed. My father and his team of helpers used to do this at such locations as Town Hall steps in all weathers. He did this until he developed his final and fatal illness, acute miliary tuberculosis.

It was to be many years before I was to appreciate both the effects of these experiences upon me as an individual, and his influence upon me as a role model. I last saw him a day or two before he died, when he expressed his delight on learning that I had won a scholarship to grammar school and urged me to make the best of the opportunity. He was extremely frail at the time, weighing only six stones, but his eyes were bright and his mind crystal clear. It is quite astonishing to me to see how society has changed for the better, for I see no evidence of the grinding poverty of those days in Britain today.

My mother was a staunch Anglican of the High Church variety, and my brothers and I were boat boys, choristers and servers in our local church. We attended Sunday School and church services regularly. During all those difficult days she laboured incessantly, whilst nursing my father, to keep her family clothed, fed and warm. Fortunately, she was an excellent and thrifty manager and a splendid cook who constantly seemed to be able to produce nutritious and filling meals from minuscule amounts of food.

My mouth still waters when I recall her suet puddings, pies and cooked vegetables. She was not so successful at keeping us warm for at that time the houses were cold and draughty and fires were seldom lit in more than one room. Life in those days was hard for ordinary folk, like us, who did not possess refrigerators, washing machines, gas or electric cookers, hot water systems, central heating, double glazing or even, on occasions, flush toilets. Coal or coke was the everyday fuel and from a young age I used to break up coal into pieces of manageable size and chop up kindling wood for her use. Washing clothes was done in a coal fired copper boiler, they were scrubbed on a board and lifted out with a stick. They were wrung out using a large mangle with wooden rollers, and I recall standing on a box whilst turning the handle. Truly a woman's work was never done, for the stoves had to be blackleaded, the steps covered in white or red ochre, the tiled floors scrubbed and the brasses polished. Whilst there was usually a grate in every room, those in the bedrooms were minuscule and a fire was only lit in them when someone was ill.

We did not have a bathroom and were bathed in a

galvanised tub which hung on a hook on the wall outside the kitchen door when not in use. Hot water was transferred into it from the copper with a wood handled baler which was also used to empty it when the ablutions were finished. Even when a fire was lit in the living room only the hearth close to it was warm, sometimes too warm, and the remainder of the room was cold. A kettle was usually kept bubbling on the hob whenever a fire was alight.

As my mother also had to cope with my father's illnesses and repeated absences it is small wonder that she aged markedly during this period and was constantly tired and depressed.

Despite all the problems that I have described my memories of these times are happy ones. I loved playing in the countryside and fishing in the stream for tiddlers. I was a foolhardy tree climber and was often seen sitting reading high up in a tree, overhanging the Great Western Railway line to the West Country. For a number of years I attended a small Church of England Primary School, All Saints at Bourne Hill on the outskirts of Maidenhead in Berkshire. We had to walk a couple of miles to get to school in all weathers, and I often bowled a hoop or whipped a top as I walked to keep warm in the winter. We used horse chestnuts to play 'conkers', bowled alleys (glass marbles) and flipped cigarette cards against each other, played football and ran in cross country races or paper chases in our spare time. Unlike today, parents never thought that we were in any danger during these unescorted and unsupervised activities, for this was a society of unlocked doors and open windows. Various travelling salesmen such as milkmen, fruiterers, butchers, fishmongers and Corona men used to read the note on the kitchen table, leave the goods which had been ordered, take the cost from the monies left beside it and leave the change!

Television had only just been invented and had yet to be introduced into the home. We did not possess one of the newfangled wind up gramophones. I can recall my father constructing a crystal wireless set with a cat's whisker and my excitement when it worked. Later I used to take accumulators to the local garage to be charged. I also used to walk a mile each way to a farm to collect milk in a special can before going to school each day. The headmaster at All Saints School was a Mr Welch who was very tall and his deputy was Miss Jones who was extremely thin. They were both outstandingly good teachers and pupils of the school regularly obtained four or five of the twelve scholarships for grammar schools which were available locally each year. It was their practice to enter pupils for the examinations at the age of ten years, in order to gain experience which proved invaluable when they took the examination again at the normal age of eleven years. Unbeknown to them my father, who was often confined to bed by illness, spent many hours coaching me for the examinations with the result that not only did I obtain a place at grammar school, at my first attempt at the age of ten years, but I was also awarded free books and free school uniform, which in view of the family circumstances was singularly fortunate.

Sadly my father died within days of the results being announced, whilst I spent the rest of my schooldays as the youngest pupil in the class. My poor mother, exhausted by her exertions looking after a dying husband and three small children, had a mental and physical breakdown. Only then did her family come to her aid, taking her and my two younger brothers into their homes in London.

As my scholarship was not transferable until I had successfully completed at least one year at grammar school, I was fostered informally and lived with a newly wed young couple who had moved into the rented house next door to the one in which my father had died. They were kindly folk and looked after me very well but quite naturally, they had other priorities and I was a very lonely little boy. After some months my mother had recovered sufficiently to act as housekeeper in her brother's practice premises. When he and his family moved to Winchmore Hill she set about creating a home for her family, arranged for my scholarship to be transferred and sent for me. I enjoyed my time at Maidenhead County Boys School despite being the youngest boy in the school and looked down upon by some of the sons of fee paying parents.

In Harringay I found my mother working as hard as ever to look after us. Her pay was meagre to say the least and she worked extremely long hours for it. She was old fashioned enough to make it clear to me that I was now the man of the family despite my tender years and that whilst she welcomed all the help that I was able to give, my first duty was to take full advantage of the educational opportunities available to me. She had obtained a place for me at Glendale Grammar School, a co-educational establishment situated in Wood Green, close to its border with Palmers Green, several miles from my home. Fortunately, the Number 29 tram took me from door to door. Later it was replaced by the Number 629 trolleybus. I enjoyed my time there and made good academic progress except in French at which I was hopeless. To this day I remain a poor linguist! I played football and participated in all the social activities at the school which did not require finance. The Headmaster was a Mr Dyment who was dyspeptic and very much against smoking. Thus when all the School Prefects, including the School Captain, were caught smoking in the cycle shed, he expelled all of them at once. Unfortunately for him, there were not enough sixth formers left to replace the expellees and so, although I was only in the fifth form and was a year younger than my classmates, I found myself a very immature Prefect. In order to prove that I was manly, when I patently was not, I joined those who smoked regularly in the cycle shed. Fortunately I was never caught. I never enjoyed the experience and abandoned the practice as soon as it had served its purpose.

War clouds had been gathering and we were informed that the whole school was to be evacuated. On September 3rd 1939, the day that war was declared, my brother, Alan, and I were amongst those transported to the country. With our schoolmates we were taken by bus to Halstead in Essex whilst my mother and youngest brother, John, went to Much Haddam, quite a distance away. Unfortunately, we should have been taken to Halstead in Kent and so by the time that we arrived all the billets offered by the local residents had been taken up. After many hours of waiting, the Council Billeting Officer took us around the town knocking on the doors of other houses and forcing the occupants to accept us into their homes. Many of these folk had not offered to house evacuees for very good reasons, and so the next few months were a period during which we were moved from home to home, sometimes together, sometimes apart. A first class recipe for making children feel unwanted! This was my matriculation year and so I was pleased when arrangements were made for us to be taught in a local church hall.

This was the period of inaction known as the 'phoney war' and over the next few months many children went back to London, a process speeded by the odd German bomb being jettisoned over Essex. A situation developed in which most of the pupils were in London and most of the teachers were in Halstead, and so the latter were moved back to London. My brother and I had no home in London to go to and so, with a minority of other pupils, we were sent to Earl's Colne Grammar School, for two or three months. As the Blitz began the school was evacuated for a second time, this time to Newquay in Cornwall.

My unfortunate mother had successfully applied for a post in Halstead so as to be near my brother and I, but on taking it up found that we had gone to Cornwall. She spent the rest of the war acting as Matron of a hostel for problem evacuee children. I was billeted in a small private hotel run by two elderly maiden ladies, the Misses Buck, together with about thirty girls from East Ham, whilst my brother lived with a family about half a mile away. We both attended Newquay County Boys School where the Headmaster, Mr Widgery, immediately appointed me a Prefect. He and the Science teacher, Dr Roberts, realising that I had been preparing to take the General Schools Certificate Examinations of London University, and that their pupils were to take the Oxford and Cambridge Examinations, went to great pains to arrange for me to have suitable instruction in certain subjects, which were not common to the two examinations. This they did by utilising the goodwill and services of teachers in other schools evacuated to the town. I was, and still am, a hopeless linguist and after having special coaching only managed to obtain a mark of 27% in French, in the mock matriculation examination. Everyone else was horrified as I had to obtain a pass in a modern language in order to gain exemption from the matriculation examination. On the other hand, I was delighted with my mark as it was at least 20% better than any mark in French that I had ever obtained before. My language coach, an elderly lady named Miss Ireland, who invariably wore a cameo on a black band around her neck, redoubled her efforts and my homework. I took the examinations in the Bristol Hotel, which overlooked the Tolcarne Beach, and had been taken over by the young ladies of Benenden School from Kent. When I succeeded in obtaining matriculation exemption with a pass in French, albeit at Lower Standard, Miss Ireland, an Oxford graduate of the old school, told me that she had always felt that there was something seriously wrong with the Godless University of Gower Street and that my result had confirmed her views.

The next two years passed quickly. I swam in and out of the harbour every day, played football for both house and school, joined the Local Defence Volunteers when they were set up. They later became the 11th Battalion (The Chough Battalion) of the Duke of Cornwall's Light Infantry, Home Guard. At school I studied for a Mathematics based Higher Schools Certificate. There was one major hiccup. My brother, Alan, broke his leg and spent six weeks in traction in the local Cottage Hospital. I decided not to tell my mother until he had recovered as there was absolutely nothing that she could do about it other than worry. We both were, and are, notoriously bad correspondents and she insisted that we wrote to her each week before she would send us our pocket money, which was six old pennies each per week. This gave us a problem for my brother found it difficult to write whilst lying flat on his back in traction.

Fortunately, it was my custom to send her a postcard each week bearing the same legend 'Dear Mum, I am alive and well. Please send pocket money by return of post'. I merely substituted 'we are' for 'I am' and we both signed it. With great determination Alan managed to do this only to be told regularly in her letters that he should write his own card and improve his handwriting!

Although separated from our family by the length of the country we were both very happy in Cornwall for our stay there was the longest period of tranquillity that either of us had ever experienced. We became more Cornish than the Cornish and spoke with a heavy regional accent, so much so that when I went back to London I was immediately called 'Cousin Jack' and found that nobody could understand anything that I was saying.

I was fortunate enough to win a scholarship which enabled me to study either law, medicine, dentistry or veterinary science, and sought advice as to which profession I should enter. My first choice was to become a barrister, but I was advised that having no connections with the law I would probably starve if I did so, advice that was most likely correct at the time. I decided that I would rather treat people than animals but could not make my mind up between medicine and dentistry. Having always loved using my hands I did not want to be a general medical practitioner but wondered if I would find job satisfaction in dentistry. By pure chance I discovered that under the Aegis of the Royal Colleges it was possible to do a combined course in both disciplines leading to qualification in both, in six years in the London Medical and Dental Schools. My scholarship was for four years and with the naiveté and optimism of youth I wrote to the authorities explaining my dilemma and inquiring whether they would finance me for six years so that I could undertake the combined course. To their eternal credit they agreed to do so and I sought and obtained a place at the Royal Dental Hospital of London School of Dental Surgery to read for the diplomas of the Royal Colleges of Physicians and Surgeons. As this was my uncle's Alma Mater I gave his name as a referee without asking him if I could do so. Only when contacted by the school did he learn of my academic progress and career plans. He was delighted and gave me his encouragement and practical help by arranging for me to live in his practice premises on my own. At this time my elderly maternal grandparents lived next door and promised to keep an eye on me. Very excited I moved to London, an extremely gauche, countrified, religious and narrow minded seventeen year old, ignoring the bombing and knowing nothing of the rockets that were to follow. Alan was left in Cornwall on his own and my mother and youngest brother were in Halstead.

## Chapter Two

# Dental Studies

I WELL REMEMBER being frightened of the minimal traffic as I crossed the road in Leicester Square to enter the Royal. Behind me stood the bombed out shell of the old Archbishop Tennyson School on the corner of Irvine Street. In front of me lay my new life and a number of problems. The first of these was that nobody could understand a word that I said because of my broad Cornish accent. The second was to discover that I had studied the wrong subjects and so could not gain exemption from the pre-medical examination, and the third was to learn that the combined course had been discontinued for the duration of the war!

The Royal was the oldest institution of its kind in the British Commonwealth having been founded in 1858 to train students taking the LDS RCS (Eng) diploma which had just been established by the Royal College of Surgeons. The building that I entered was the third premises that the school occupied and the first purpose built dental hospital in the country. It was opened in 1901 and was in constant use until it closed in 1985. It was the first institution in Europe to provide professional training and scientific education for dentists.

There was a tremendous atmosphere about the place which was engendered and maintained by a number of long serving staff. The first of these was Jack Knights who was porter and head porter from 1924 to 1964 and was a great character. It was he who greeted me as I entered its portals for the first time. He took pity on me and we became great friends. Miss Helen M. Duncan, known to everyone as 'Nellie', joined the staff of the hospital in 1919 and was appointed the first school secretary in 1932. She served in that capacity until her retirement in 1948. A Scotswoman of austere appearance and strong old fashioned views she spoke with a strong Scottish accent which became more marked each year that she lived in England. Despite this it was she who pointed out to me that my broad Cornish accent would have to go if I wished to succeed in my studies. The hospital was, of course, a voluntary hospital dependent upon charitable contributions and was run most efficiently and well by Mr W.J. Ickeringill, an accountant, who served as Secretary Superintendent from 1938 to 1961. He was assisted in his task by one lady almoner, who was the first woman I had ever seen with coloured streaks in her hair, and one office junior in her teens. He could have taught the managers of our over administered and over politicised NHS hospitals today a thing or two about both economy and efficiency!

Within thirty minutes of my entering the premises Nellie ushered me into the office of the longest serving Dean of the Institution in its entire history, Professor Harry Stobie, who served in that capacity from 1920 until his death in 1948. During the war he also spent half his time serving as a Brigadier in the Army Medical Service. This delightful, outstanding, talented, benevolent and able man informed me of my academic situation and asked me which of the two courses I wished to pursue. He told me that whilst the Royal was staying in London, if I chose to read medicine I would be transferred to Guy's, which had been evacuated to

Tunbridge Wells. Having been told that I had twenty minutes to make my mind up I tried to contact my Uncle by telephone, with Jack Knight's help, but failed to do so. As I had accommodation arranged, had found my way from it to the hospital by bus and the Tube, liked the little that I had seen of the Royal and had not the faintest idea where Tunbridge Wells was, I chose dentistry. Had I chosen to read medicine on that occasion I feel sure that I would have had an entirely different career.

Arrangements were quickly made for me to study at a famous crammers, Carlyle and Gregson (Jimmies) in Earl's Court, where Winston Churchill had been a student decades earlier. Under their expert tutelage I completed the two year course in Physics, Chemistry and Biology in four months starting from scratch. I scraped through the pre-medical examination, despite having no real understanding of the subjects, and commenced my studies proper at the Royal. The London Blitz began in September 1940 and on the 17th October the Royal was damaged by a land mine. Repairs were effected but after the windows had been blown out several times, the broken glass was replaced by boarding. This had the effect of making us dependent upon artificial light, often of inadequate quality, when treating patients. At the time of my arrival there were only a total of one hundred and ten students in all years combined in the Dental School, and so we lived extremely busy lives. We attended the Royal Free Hospital Medical School for Women to study Anatomy and Physiology, being taught by three members of their Consultant Staff, the Misses Barry, Sands and Hewer. They were excellent teachers and I used to attend Miss Barry's operating sessions in the basement of the Royal Homeopathic Hospital in Queen Square, and make myself as useful as I could. We were taught dental mechanics by two dentists registered under a grandfather clause in the 1921 Dentists Act: 'Uncle' New and 'Gillie' Gilson who were both characters although entirely different in nature. 'Uncle' was very serious and dedicated to his job, while it was well known that 'Gillie' liked a drink especially with students of like mind. Most of the academic staff, who were mainly honorary and part timers, were away serving in the armed forces. They were replaced by a number of distinguished colleagues who came out of retirement to help by teaching us on a part time and ad hoc basis. They served the hospital and school on a voluntary basis and earned their living in private practice. Two distinguished Oral Surgeons, B.W. Fickling and Desmond Greer Walker, who were running maxillofacial Units in the Emergency Medical Service also attended the Royal regularly. Many lectures were given either during the lunch break or in the early evening, the order in which they were given being determined by the availability of the teachers in question. As the curriculum is planned in a sequential manner this meant that we often did courses before attending the foundation course upon which they were based but somehow we managed. The vast clinical experience of such men as S.A. Riddett, 'Frankie' Coleman, 'Charlie' Packham, Cyril Bowdler Henry, W.E. Earle (Bill) and Lionel 'Spike' Hardwick saw us through.

They were all West End practitioners of the highest order and leading lights in the profession. We could not have had better role models. As most of the qualified dental surgeons in the country were serving in the armed forces and dental disease was of epidemic proportions the Royal was literally besieged by patients seeking relief from pain. We arrived in the mornings to find literally hundreds of people queuing from the Patients' Entrance at the back of the building alongside the hospital and into Leicester Square.

Another wonderful Cockney character, Bill Gale, was employed full time to control the influx of patients which he did with unfailing courtesy and compassion day in and day out. To cope with this emergency service all clinical students were required to work in the clinics of the hospital every morning and afternoon for five and a half days each week. In the majority of cases the dental diseases were so advanced that teeth had to be extracted and many patients who had never had any form of dental care required multiple extractions or even the removal of all their natural teeth, a dental clearance, but more of this later.

Students and staff shared fire watching duties and several incendiary devices which landed on the premises were dealt with effectively. We also took turns to serve in the First Aid Centre at Charing Cross Hospital, in which we studied Medicine and Surgery under the guidance of Dr Hamilton and Mr Zieve, respectively. Others, including me, also served in the Home Guard. I had transferred into Number 13 platoon, D Company, 28th Battalion the Middlesex Regiment which was based in barracks in Wood Green. By this time we had been equipped with American Springfield rifles and Browning machine guns of First World War vintage, as well as primitive mortars such as the Blacker Bombard, Mills hand grenades and petrol bombs. I trained as an armourer and reached the dizzy rank of Corporal.

Morale was high in London, despite the bombing and the V1 and V2 rockets. We were all companions in misfortune and people went out of their way to help each other. Women could walk around in the blackout without the fear of being attacked and regularly did so. Hundreds of people of all ages slept on metal bunks on the platforms of underground stations every night to shelter from the bombing, and the Voluntary Services did whatever they could to ease their lot. I used to pass them on my journeys to and from the Royal.

Every home had been supplied with an Anderson air raid shelter which comprised of a series of corrugated iron sheets which one assembled using the bolts provided and placed in a hole dug for the purpose in the garden and then covered with the earth which had been dug out. One was supposed to sleep in the shelter every night and cower in it when the air raid warnings sounded during the day. Not surprisingly, few people did so for long for these structures were cold, draughty and damp and ill suited to human habitation. I certainly preferred to take the chance of meeting my maker in my own bed, in my own room, despite the windows being blown out once or twice. Later the Morrison shelter was issued. It consisted of a sheet metal base and heavy metal flat roof which was supported by four two-sided struts, one at each corner. The sides of this contraption were metal meshwork. This shelter was erected in a ground floor room of the house and as one could put a mattress inside it, it was a much more acceptable sleeping place. Every citizen was issued with a gas mask and instructed in its use. We carried them with us at all times usually in a tin to which was attached a shoulder strap. Fortunately we never had to use them, except in practice, and most of us regarded them as an encumbrance and a nuisance.

The radio and the cinema were the main forms of entertainment, and became part of one's life. I used to go to the Finsbury Park Astoria cinema regularly as the programmes changed weekly. This was a huge building beautifully decorated and lit internally as a Moorish Palace.

When funds permitted I also went to the Music Hall, usually either the Finsbury Park or Wood Green Empire. There I saw such artists as Florrie Ford, Nellie Wallace, Elsie and Doris Waters, Sid Field, 'Fats' Waller and many others in person. The radio programmes were repetitive and often featured the same small group of performers. Music While You Work, Reginald Foort and Sandy Macpherson playing the BBC Cinema Organ, Henry Hall and the BBC Dance Band, Carol Gibbons and the Savoy Hotel Orpheans, Ambrose and Ted Heath and their orchestras. Tommy Handley in ITMA (It's That Man Again), Arthur Askey and 'Stinker' Murdoch, Ted Ray, Tommy Trinder and Flanagan and Allen and the Crazy Gang kept us laughing, often at ourselves.

My other social pastime was ballroom dancing which was extremely popular in those days. Dances and dance schools were everywhere to be found. The latter were often part time activities and run by younger people who, like me, were in so called 'Reserved Occupations', doing what was considered to be essential work for society. One of my friends and his wife ran such an institution on weekday evenings and provided instruction for the bronze, silver and gold medal examinations. Their main problem was a severe shortage of suitable male partners for the girl students to dance with in practice, and even more importantly in the actual examinations. They asked me to help them in this way and provided me with the necessary instruction free of charge. This I did one or two evenings each week and I soon lost count of the number of medal examinations that I participated in, although never as a candidate.

Towards the end of my studies I met Heather who was destined to transform my life. As I have already mentioned the Royal was besieged by patients seeking relief from pain. Every final year student was required to serve as an emergency dresser for one day each week and we worked in pairs. Our duty was to provide treatment for those patients in whom tooth extraction was not indicated. As most of these patients had filthy neglected mouths and many also had a gum infection, then called AUG (Acute Ulcerative Gingivitis), which is characterised by an offensive foul odour on the breath which made diagnosis possible at a range of some yards, this was not a popular assignment. AUG was endemic in the trenches in the 1914-1918 war, when it was called 'Trench Mouth'. On occasions it laid low companies or even battalions of soldiers, causing major problems, for the Army Dental Corps was not formed until 1924 and the small number of dentists then serving on the General List were very few and far between.

This unattractive clinical situation was bad enough but it was made worse by the fact that the number of patients was such as to ensure that the Emergency Dressers seldom, if ever, got a lunch break and worked continuously from 9 a.m. until the early evening.

As food rationing was severe, even basic foods such as bread being rationed, we did not have the advantage of starting the day with a good breakfast. Antibiotic therapy had yet to be introduced and so we spent the day removing gross decay and inserting sedative dressings in the tooth cavities, applying medicaments such as Chromic Acid and Hydrogen Peroxide to ulcerated gums, removing tartar and inserting sedative packing between teeth, whilst getting thirstier and thirstier and hungrier and hungrier.

On the day in question my spirits were rising as my colleague and I had matters under control to such an extent

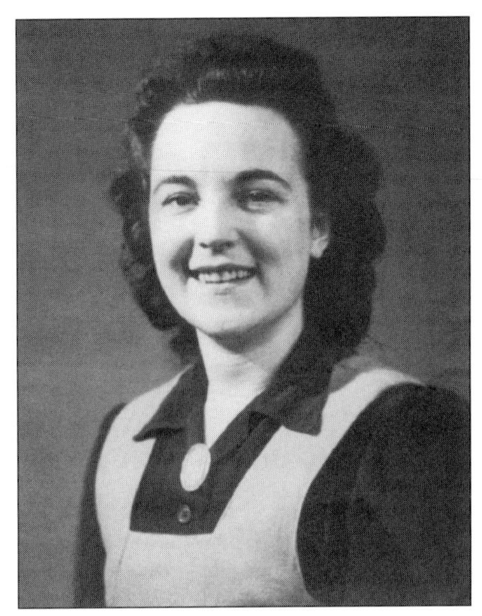

*Heather and I at time that we met.*

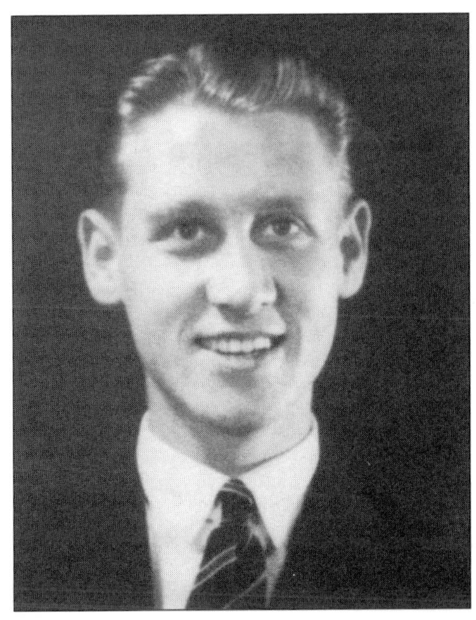

that we looked like getting a lunch break for the first time in weeks. But it was not to be, for just as I was clearing up to go, another yellow casualty card was presented to me with the whispered comment that 'she is a nurse who has just come off duty'. With no more ado a very attractive Red Cross VAD nurse in uniform was ushered in and informed me that a filling in a front tooth recently inserted by a private dentist, had been lost and that the tooth was causing her considerable pain. Examination revealed that a large amount of decay (caries) was still present in the cavity, and so I removed most of this and inserted a sedative dressing which soon relieved the pain. I then told the patient to make an appointment to have a permanent restoration inserted at some future date, thinking as I did so that I still had time for a sandwich and a glass of milk before starting work again. The lady then asked me when I thought that I would be able to fill the tooth permanently. I explained that it would not be me who did this as I was nearing the end of my training and trying to complete the treatment of all my existing patients, before taking my Final Examinations. At this she became very agitated and demanded that I give her an appointment remarking that she felt that people who started jobs should finish them! I was very annoyed at her attitude and tried to explain the difficulties under which we were working. An argument about the demerits of the system developed and my chances of a lunch break diminished rapidly. Finally, in order to get the time to have a glass of milk, as I could hear the sound of new patients coming up the stairs, I gave her the appointment and we parted on bad terms.

Little did I know the significance of that hasty decision for when she kept that appointment and I examined her whole mouth I was appalled by what I found. Most of her teeth had been recently filled so poorly that I considered that every restoration in her mouth would have to be replaced if her teeth were to be saved, an opinion soon confirmed by the teachers on duty, Bill Earle and Spike Hardwick. My consternation was nothing compared to hers when she was informed of our opinion for she had spent many hours having the work done by a well known, and very expensive, fashionable dentist in Harley Street. She was so distressed that I suggested that I give her another appointment so that she could decide what she wanted to do. This she did and on her return she asked me to do whatever was necessary to enable her to keep her teeth. In the circumstances I felt duty bound to take on this commitment despite having a full and closed list of so called 'private' patients. During the next few months I saw her whenever it was possible to squeeze her in, often two or three times each week. This was hardly the best way to get to know one another for in those days, and in wartime conditions the engines, drills and local anaesthetic solutions available for use were primitive by today's standards. She was an excellent patient and we were able to save all her teeth except for one molar which, unfortunately, I had to extract as we had no equipment or facilities for molar endodontics at that time. I am happy to say that she never lost another tooth and that when she died more than fifty years later some of the restorations that I inserted at that time were still in situ.

During this period of treatment we got to know each other and became friends. This surprised everyone, and especially me for it soon became obvious to both of us that we were complete opposites and had virtually nothing in common. As previously described I was gauche and unworldly and intolerant of behaviour of which I disapproved, and had no hesitation in passing judgement on others and letting them know my opinion. A non-smoking teetotaller, I had never set foot in a theatre in which a ballet, an opera or a play had been performed. Without realising it at the time, I was both a bigot and a prig. Heather's background could not have been more different from mine. Her father, whom I never met, was a cartographer employed by the Ordnance Survey Department who, in his spare time, developed the Foldex system of maps which was so popular with motorists for many years. He came from Menhenniot, near Liskeard and after marrying the village belle, Winifred Mary, of St Stephen's near Saltash was transferred to London. Heather was the elder of his two daughters who were the light of his life. He took them everywhere, the Houses of Parliament, Museums, State Occasions etc. Unfortunately he developed cancer in his early forties and underwent major surgery in St Mark's Hospital, which sustained a direct hit during night bombing a few hours later. He was dug out of the wreckage and survived for about a year. Heather was by this time a Civil Servant having gained a scholarship to a prestigious Public School, the Burlington, and obtaining a very high ranking in the Civil Service Examinations. She was posted to the Air Ministry where she gained rapid promotion in the war years. Her duties brought her into contact with many aircrew, including 'Cats Eyes' Cunningham and Guy Gibson VC, when they were posted to the Air Ministry in between tours of active service operations. These airmen knew the risks that they were taking and so had a very active social life despite wartime limitations. When she wasn't working either in her job or as a VAD in the National Temperance Hospital in Tottenham Court Road or the Leicester Square

Underground Air Raid Shelter, Heather took part in this social round, partying in hotels, nightclubs and restaurants. She became engaged more than once to aircrew but they and many of her other friends were killed on active service. When we met she was just coming to terms with yet another loss, drinking half a bottle of black market whisky and smoking twenty cigarettes a day. A very sophisticated lady!

As at that time I was an impecunious teetotaller and as she never at any time liked drinking alone her intake of alcohol dropped dramatically. She gave up smoking overnight when I told her that I did not relish kissing 'Fag Ash Lil'! During the rest of her life she never smoked another cigarette although freely admitting that she had the urge to do so quite frequently. With my blessing she occasionally indulged herself by smoking a small cigar after enjoying a good dinner.

During one of our later treatment sessions an appointments clerk came up to me and said that a young lady named Ivy had telephoned to say that she could not accompany me to the dance on Saturday, as she had influenza. As soon as my ministrations would allow, Heather asked me about Ivy and the dance. I explained that Ivy was one of the several dance partners, that I was helping to prepare for their medal examinations, and that the dance in question was merely a Student Hop at the Hospital Sports Pavilion at Colindale, being run by the Soccer Club of which I was the Secretary. At the end of the session she said that she had never been to a University do of any kind. She went on to say that if I was short of a partner for the evening she would love to come along provided that she could bring her schoolfriend, Kay, who worked in South Africa House. I knew that my friend, Albert Kamsler, had no partner for the evening so I invited him to make up a foursome and we all went to our first social occasion together, which was not an entire success as both the ladies had something to learn about ballroom dancing. Nevertheless we all enjoyed ourselves and agreed to meet again. This we did and spent many happy hours in the 'Gods' (Uppermost Balcony) in the Sadler's Wells and other theatres where I acquired my lifelong love of opera and ballet.

Despite the ad hoc arrangements, or perhaps because of them, I completed all the courses required to take the Final Examinations before I reached my twenty-first birthday, and so was too young to be admitted to the examinations. It was decided that I should spend a few months working as a Student House Officer at the Ministry of Pensions Hospital at Stoke Mandeville in Buckinghamshire. My chief was Desmond Greer Walker, a genial, friendly and talented Irish oral surgeon, who was also on the Consultant Staff of both the Royal and the Middlesex Hospitals. It was a wonderful experience for me, for Desmond and his plastic surgery colleague, Mr Pomfret Kilner, were making great advances in the treatment of war wounds, especially maxillofacial injuries and burns. A highlight of the week was the Combined Clinic when they were joined by a Professor of Anatomy and a Professor of Bacteriology, and devised new approaches to treatment and reviewed the results of their previous endeavours. Dr Ludwig Gutman was undertaking his pioneering studies on the management of spinal injuries in the other wing of the hospital, work which was to transform the lives of thousands of such patients and lead to the foundation of the paraolympics, and it was a privilege to learn from him. Many years later it was my delight to nominate him for an Honorary degree in the University of

Newcastle upon Tyne. All in all it was a most exciting and rewarding experience to be in such a centre of excellence, and I returned to the Royal to take my finals full of enthusiasm for dentistry, my chosen profession. After qualification I was appointed House Surgeon in the Children's and Orthodontic Department at the Royal and worked under the supervision of Clifford Ballard who went on to transform orthodontics from a mechanical trade into a biomechanical clinical science in his capacity of Professor and Founder Head of the Department of Orthodontics at the Postgraduate Institute based at the Eastman Dental Hospital, Gray's Inn Road. He was a most original thinker who collaborated widely with workers in allied disciplines such as biometrics and speech therapy.

The present day orthodontic service of the National Health Service owes much to his endeavours. A workaholic with extremely high standards and a sharp tongue, he was widely regarded as being moody and difficult to work for. However, I got on extremely well with him, learned much from him and enjoyed his friendship throughout his long and fruitful career.

I was then appointed Senior House Surgeon and was answerable to the part time Consultant Staff for the standards of both in-patient and out-patient care in co-operation with the Medical Registrar, an awesome responsibility for which I was paid less than three pounds per week, live out!

Thus it was necessary for me to work in my uncle's practice in the evenings, weekends and on bank holidays. In fact I lived on the monies that I earned in practice and saved all my hospital earnings in order to buy an engagement ring. By this time Heather had taken me home to meet her sister, Sheila, and her mother, Winifred Mary. The latter's

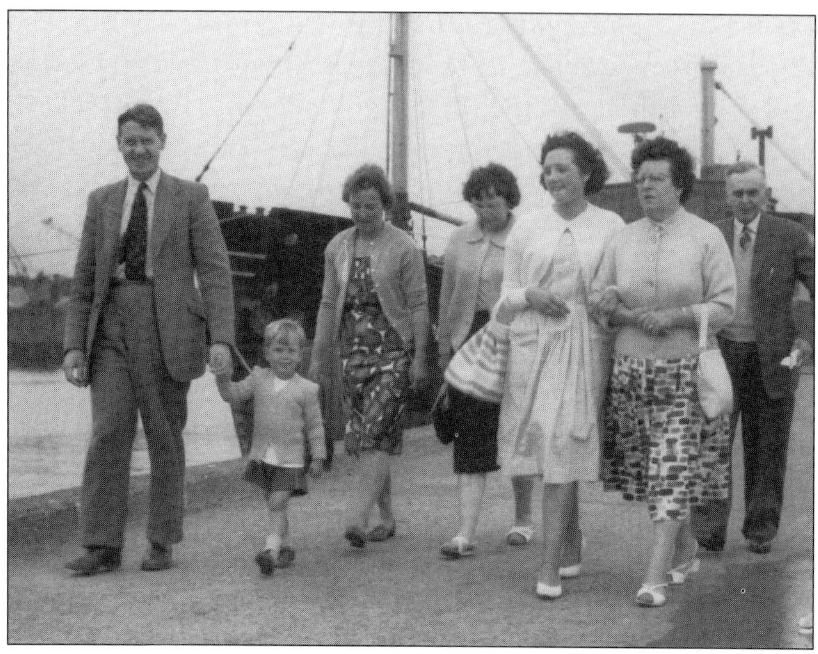

*With Heather's family. Timothy John holds my hand whilst Heather is beside her sister Sheila whose daughter Linda, our god-daughter, holds the arm of my beloved mother-in-law Winifred Mary, whose husband Alf, Heather's stepfather, brings up the rear.*

comment after our first meeting was obviously related to my impoverished appearance for she first told Heather that she thought I seemed to be a nice person but then went on to enquire where had she found me!

Although widowed young Winifred Mary was a lively person who maintained a very happy home in which friends, even impecunious ones, were always welcomed and lavishly entertained despite wartime and post war limitations. Unfortunately neither my mother nor my uncle took to Heather as they thought that she was far too sophisticated and worldly wise for me. They were concerned that she might influence me to reject their plans for me which were, in essence, that after demobilisation I join my Uncle's general practice as an assistant, with a view to an eventual partnership, and marry the young lady of their choice.

The war in Europe ended in July 1945 and the Royal students and staff, including me, being based in Leicester Square, were well placed to participate in and enjoy to the full the Victory in Europe Celebrations in London on the 8th and 9th of July.

It was decided to revive the pre-war practice of holding a formal prize giving ceremony and conversazione at the Royal. The Minister of Health, a Conservative named Willinck, was invited to present the prizes and give the address, and he agreed to do so. However, in the first post-war General Election a Labour Government was elected to power and the Welsh radical Socialist, Aneurin Bevan, was appointed Minister of Health. As the invitation had been made to the office and not to the individual there was much fluttering in the dovecotes of the ultra conservative Royal. My dilemma was a different one for I was informed by the Dean's office that, having qualified, I must wear a dark suit and an LDS RCS (Eng) gown when collecting the several prizes that I had won during my studies. Clothes were rationed during the war and I only possessed one dark suit, the trousers of which were threadbare and frayed, and did not possess an LDS gown or know where to get one. My friend the porter, Jack Knight, found one for me, I know not from where, and his wife kindly washed and ironed it for me. I solved the problem of the frayed trouser bottoms with the aid of an iron and a surgical scalpel the night before the Prize giving.

Aneurin Bevan appeared in a gingery brown suit with a red tie, gave out the prizes in a delightful manner and spoke

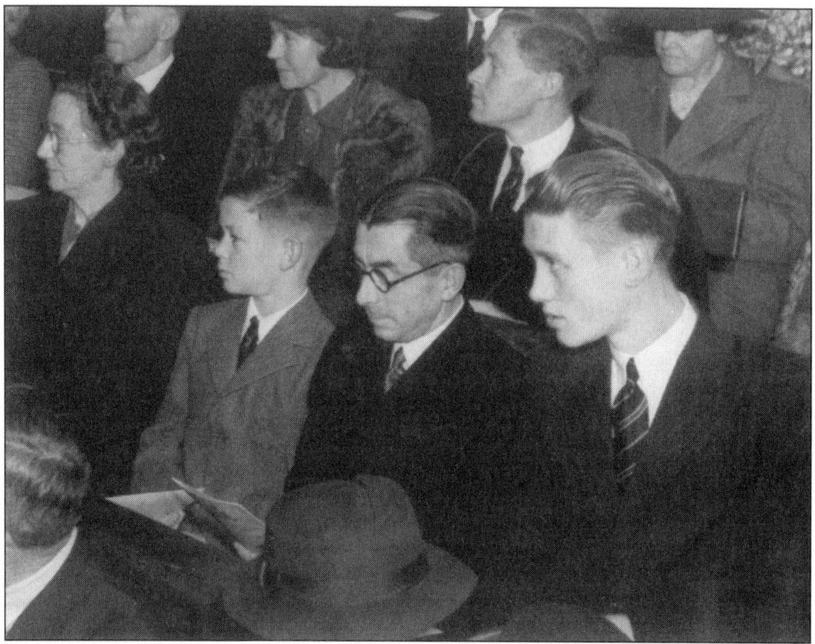

*At the Royal Dental prizegiving. From left to right, my mother, my cousin John and Uncle Sid.*

to an obviously hostile audience without turning a hair. I admired him tremendously both as a man and as a politician, and was very impressed with the way in which he handled the introduction of the National Health Service. Unfortunately our only other meeting was during his terminal illness.

During and immediately after the war the activities of both qualified dentists and dental students were controlled by a Dental Manpower Committee, and dental students were not allowed to join the armed forces until qualification. House officers were only given their War Emergency Commissions after completing their hospital appointments. Having always loved the sea I was very keen to join the Royal Navy but unfortunately at the time my house officer appointments ended there were no vacancies in that service, and so, much against my wishes, I received an Army War Emergency Commission in the rank of Lieutenant.

Just before reporting for duty in No 306 Army Dental Centre, Marlborough Lines, Aldershot, in early December 1946, I proposed to Heather and was accepted, much to the consternation of my family and the astonishment of hers!

## Chapter Three

# Army Days

I MUST CONFESS that I joined the Army in low spirits and with bad grace. When I arrived in Aldershot I met a very harassed and overworked Captain Lees, who having said that he was pleased to hear that I, like him, was a Royal man, told me that if I would help him deal with the rest of the dental sick parade, he would show me where I would be sleeping. Two hours later he took me to the Cambridge Hospital Mess, which at that time was peopled by very senior middle aged RAMC officers who did not exactly put out the red carpet for a mere subaltern in the then Army Dental Corps. Furthermore, the buildings were Victorian, cold and draughty, fuel was scarce and snow plentiful.

I had to walk the length of Queen's Avenue to and from the Dental Centre twice each day. During these excursions, and despite having had no formal military instruction since being in the OTC in my first grammar school, I was required to acknowledge the salutes of the numerous bodies of men marching along the Avenue, who varied from companies of airborne troops to German prisoners of war.

The daily dental sick parades were enormous and I soon discovered that their size was swollen by a number of officer cadets from Mons Barracks seeking refuge from the exhortations of R.S.M. Britten and his sidekick, C.S.M. Parnaby, whose dulcet tones could be heard from afar. Captain Lees and I and our support staff which included

Erich, the sole survivor of a German U-boat, worked flat out all day, every day to deal with the casualty load, no time being available for elective treatment. On my tenth day in the Army orders came through that I was to take over the Dental Centre at Southwood Camp at Cove, near Farnborough, Hants. I was transported to the camp together with my few possessions in a PU van and found that the Dental Centre was a wooden hut just like every other building in the camp, other than the guardroom which was brick built. It housed the Light Infantry Brigade Training Centre (LIBTC) which received all the recruits for the Somerset LI, the Duke of Cornwall's LI, the Oxon and Bucks LI, the Shropshire LI, the Kings Own Yorkshire LI and the Durham LI. The commanding officer was Brigadier Hulton Harrap DSO, late Shropshire LI and everything ran like clockwork. It was extremely fortunate for me that the DCLI were there for I was soon greeted by friends and acquaintances from my Newquay schooldays, who introduced me to military administration and customs, and made sure that nobody took advantage of my inexperience in such matters. Despite the day beginning at 6.00 a.m. with either physical training and/or a cross country run before breakfast, morale was extremely high and the standard of physical fitness impressive. Although I had played football throughout my time at the Royal, my sedentary lifestyle had taken its toll and I found it difficult to keep up with them at first. However, with the guidance and assistance of the PT instructors I was soon enjoying these sessions.

After breakfast the dental sick parade was held at 8.00 a.m. and kept me busy for much of the day. Two hundred recruits arrived every fortnight many of whom had never seen a toothbrush before they were issued with one. I was required to examine them all individually, soon after their arrival, and to chart their dental condition on induction, the record cards being filled out by my one dental clerk orderly, Corporal 'Nuggy' Fuller. The nickname 'Nuggy' was an abbreviation for 'Nuggets', for this great character, a typical Essex man, was an inveterate and lucky gambler. Indeed so successful was he that all six of the bookmakers' runners in the camp finally refused to take bets from him. His response was typical, he simply asked everyone around him, including me, to place bets for him. Having been brought up to abhor gambling I accompanied my refusal to help him with a short sermon. I need not have bothered for he continued to make much more money than I.

The dental condition of the recruits was appalling and our first task was to give instruction in oral hygiene. The next job was to extract all carious (decayed) teeth beyond repair and roots which were often abscessed, which were either causing problems or likely to do so. As they only stayed with us for six weeks training before being posted to their respective regiments, all of which were on active service, this was a challenging and demanding task. We were also required to provide elective treatment for the permanent staff of the camp which included one ATS company, largely composed of office workers and cooks.

On arrival at the Officer's Mess, I was greeted by the Mess Sergeant who told me that one of my former schoolmates had arranged for me to share a bedroom with him and another officer. I was pleased to hear this and was surprised to receive a rather frosty reception when taken to the room by the sergeant. When he had left I was in the middle of saying that I would ask for a move if that was their wish, when they burst out laughing and opened the wardrobe in which two naked ladies were standing giggling uncontrollably. I was then informed that they worked in the NAAFI and had brought cake, tea, sugar and milk for a welcoming tea, which after donning their clothes, they prepared using the coke fired Tortoise stove for the purpose.

My arrival in the Aldershot and Hants district of Southern Command had been welcomed by the officers of the AD Corps, all of whom had leave due to them. Christmas was approaching and I was told that I would be 'holding the fort' for all of them over Christmas and the New Year, including the Command Specialist. For this purpose I was posted back to the Cambridge Military Hospital. and was introduced to the Command Specialist to whom I expressed my doubts as to whether I was experienced enough to stand in for him. I was astounded to hear that he had been put in the job on the basis of his seniority in the Corps, not his training or experience, and that he had never held a house appointment in his career. My first experience of the Bugginses Turn form of promotion and advancement!

We were quite busy over the holiday period but my abiding memory of it is of being astounded at the amount of alcohol consumed by both staff and patients for I was, of course, still a teetotaller at the time, and at the size and quality of the Christmas dinner provided, for I had been on civilian rations for the entire war, and so had never seen anything like it before.

I returned to Cove and resumed duty there soon becoming part of the LIBTC. It was only after some months that I learned that I was not the first, but the fourth, dental officer attached to them, my three predecessors having been rejected by them as being unsuitable for their purposes.

Being ignorant I had just fitted into all Unit activities and not claimed any privileges or exemptions. In addition to participating in the PT training and cross country runs, I played football for the DCLI, successfully completed the cross country/hill climb motor cycle course when all subalterns in the infantry were required to do so, participated fully in the social activities and took evening classes in woodwork with the other ranks. I enjoyed life with the Light Infantry Brigade as much as my predecessors had not. I was very impressed with the success of army training and the results achieved.

On average, in each intake of two hundred, twenty were found to be unable to read and write and a further twenty to be physically unfit to undergo strenuous training. The former were sent to Primary Education Centres in which they were coached by RAEC sergeants for six weeks. At the end of this period eighteen of them returned to the LIBTC able to read and write, a sad commentary on their previous decade of schooling.

The Physical Education Centres obtained similar successes with the physically unfit. Overall it was good to see a largely nondescript group of individuals transformed into smart, bright and fit young soldiers in so short a time,

About the time that the AD Corps became the Royal Army Dental Corps the rest of the Army exchanged its ugly khaki berets for soft coloured ones. The Light Infantry had a distinctive green one and I was delighted to be presented with one such beret with the new cap badge of my corps on it, especially so as the RADC colour was always green, albeit of a different hue, except for a very short period when it was royal blue. I wore the beret with pride until directed not to do so by an irate Assistant Director of Dental Services who told me that it was an offence to wear unauthorised headwear! I am afraid that he did not see the joke when I quietly asked if he thought that Field Marshal Lord Montgomery would be put on a charge for habitually wearing a black Tank Corps beret with two cap badges on it.

The LIBTC was peopled with characters, none more so than the Provost Sergeant, Sergeant Cox, whose turn out was always perfect. He was responsible for the excellent appearance of the camp for he ensured that all necessary work was carried out promptly by the Jankers Wallahs, or minor miscreants, under his charge. When detailed for dental treatment he came to see me pleading that he was far too busy to spare the time. I sensed that he feared dental treatment but did not wish to be so indiscreet as to exercise his right to refuse it. After a little soldierly verbal sparring I agreed to cancel his appointment, a decision which ensured that the dental centre became the top priority in the camp for repairs and redecoration. His pride and joy was known throughout the camp as Cox's folly. It comprised an earth mound around the base of the flagpole at the entrance to the barracks covered with immaculate grass inlaid with the cap badges of the six regiments picked out in whitewashed stones. The result of many hours work by Jankers Wallahs it really was an impressive artefact and Sergeant Cox, with his pace stick held smartly under his arm, was often seen to be standing alongside it, a very proud man. The first problem arose when a CRE (Civilian Royal Engineer) official told him that it would have to be removed as the flagpole was hinged at its base to facilitate its painting and the folly would prevent it being lowered. Sergeant Cox nearly exploded and shouted, 'When it needs painting I will b—y paint it!' and the official beat a hasty retreat.

The second problem was the secretary of the local golf

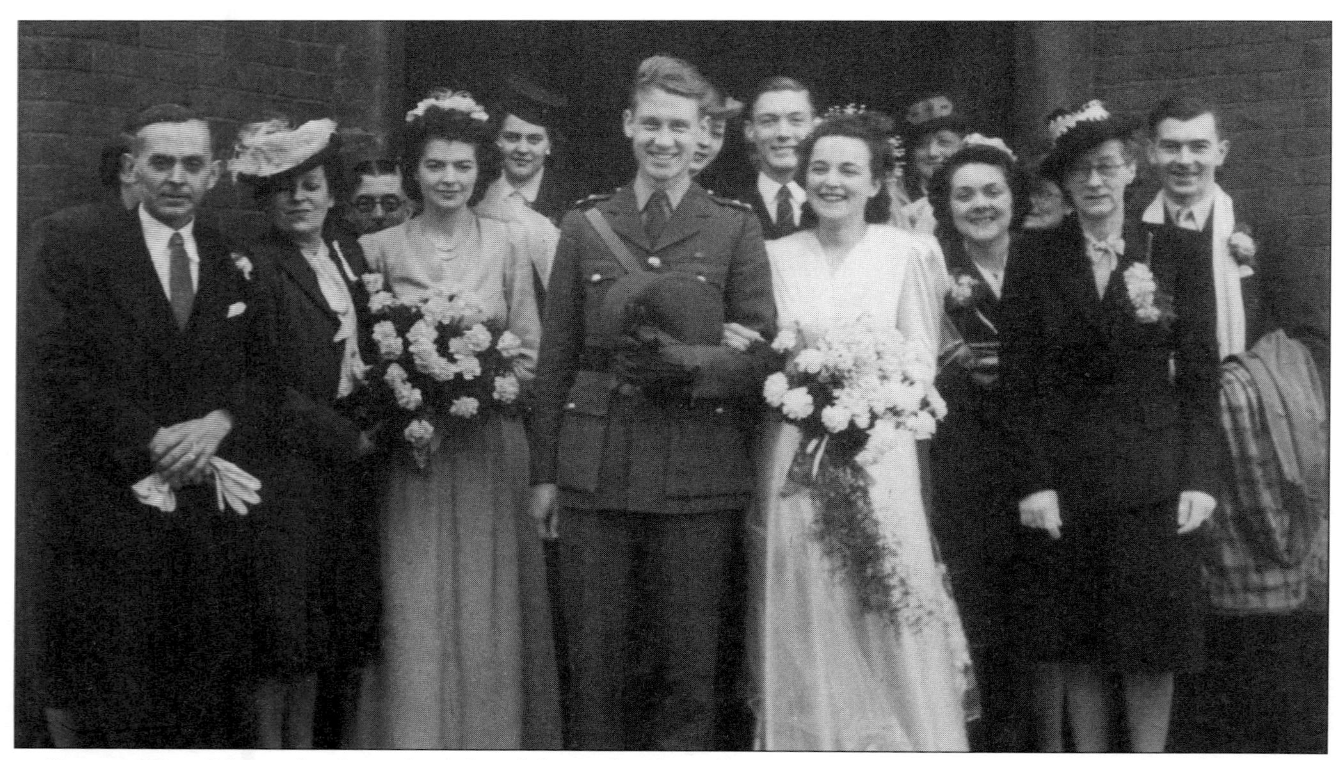

***Our wedding.** My mother is on the right whilst my brother Alan is behind us. Kay Walters, the bridesmaid, stands alongside Winifred Mary and Heather's stepfather Alf.*

club, a retired Brigadier, who came to see the Commanding Officer. He explained that whilst the golf course was not in use because of the hostilities basic maintenance was undertaken at intervals. Quite recently it had been discovered that the entire seventh green was missing. When passing the entrance to the camp he had noted the quality of the turf covering the folly and wished to enquire whether it might have something to do with the golf club's loss. Sergeant Cox was summoned to the CO's office and asked if he knew anything about the matter. Standing rigidly to attention he replied in the negative and was invited by the CO to show the golf club secretary and himself the site from which the turfs covering the folly were obtained. All three proceeded to a nearby lane where Sergeant Cox demonstrated the defects in the hedgerow created when the turfs were removed. The golf club secretary apologised profusely for his suspicions and departed. Sergeant Cox and the CO returned to the camp. As soon as they were back in his office the CO, who knew his man only too well, asked Sergeant Cox what he had done with the turfs that he had taken from the hedgerow, and standing rigidly to attention the Provost Sergeant had replied, 'Chucked 'em over the b—y hedge, sir,' thus ending the matter!

Having been notified that I was likely to be posted overseas in the near future I discussed the situation with Heather and we decided to get married without delay, against the advice of both families. This we did on April 8th 1947 at St Paul's Church, Cavendish Road, Harringay. I came home on leave the night before the day of the wedding and we had a few days honeymoon in Shanklin in the Isle of Wight before I returned to my unit.

When I got back I found that my posting had been

cancelled and that I was to stay at the LIBTC for the foreseeable future. This I did until someone in authority discovered that I had not done the Basic Officers Training Course held at the RADC depot which was then in the Cavalry Barracks in Aldershot, where the living accommodation left much to be desired. I was allowed to sleep in the LIBTC Officers Mess and commute to the course by motor cycle each day. This I did and I thoroughly enjoyed the course which was half professional and half military. My fellow students were all new entrants and so I had the advantage of having made all the administrative errors in practice during the preceding year, and passed out in top position at the end of the course.

Regular commissions had just been reintroduced in the post-war period and I was pressed to apply for one but did not do so after discussing the matter with my wife on the telephone. I returned to duty at Cove only to find that the LIBTC was moving out and relocating in excellent modern barracks in Bordon, Hants. I applied to go with them but my application was refused. They were replaced at Cove by a Royal Engineer Training Battalion whose philosophy, customs and practices were quite different. I did my best to adapt to them but must confess that I found it hard to do so and so was delighted to be transferred to Bordon after about six weeks. Little did I know what was to happen there.

The dental centre was brick built and had three dental chairs, two of which were in the same large surgery. As the lone dental officer I had the choice of which chair to use and chose one of those in the large surgery. All went well for a couple of months until a regular Major was posted to the centre and quite naturally, as I was a Captain, took over the command of it. Unfortunately he was a most unpleasant man, arrogant, opinionated, very rank conscious and a very incompetent dentist. The Corporal dental surgery assistant was first class and kept the centre in pristine condition. A delightfully cultured man who got on well with everyone. It had never occurred to me that he was gay until he became the target of much abuse and ill treatment from my colleague. Every treatment session became a nightmare for he was sadistic when treating patients and my concentration was often interrupted by screams from patients in his chair. I tried to discuss the situation with him but got short shrift.

On one day each week I attended the Military Prison at Headley Down which housed long term prisoners convicted of major crimes like murder and manslaughter. It took quite a while to get into the surgery due to the elaborate security checks. Once there those prisoners who had reported dental sick were brought in one by one, often in manacles and invariably accompanied by two or more guards. Despite the unusual circumstances I was able to treat them in exactly the same way as any other patients. I never had any trouble with them, was often politely thanked for relieving them of their symptoms and was gratified to find their numbers increasing at each visit. My colleague decided that we would undertake this duty in alternate weeks. The week after his first visit I was astounded to have no patients at all to treat. On my next visit I had two, but on the one after that I had more than twenty, far more than ever before. Some of them told my Corporal that my colleague had been performing tooth extractions and other painful procedures without anaesthetic, and on being taxed by me about it some of the guards confirmed that this was the case. Thus my 'no show' session, for it took a little while for the prisoners to learn that we were doing alternate sessions. I was incensed and went to see my colleague immediately on my return to the centre and told him of the accusations. He laughed, admitted that the allegations were true and added that he could not understand my concern for these prisoners 'were garbage' and 'a disgrace to the Army'. I told him that I was a dentist and that it was incumbent upon me to do my very best for every patient that I was privileged to treat, regardless of my personal feelings about, or, towards them. When he told me to remember that I was also an officer and was required to act as one, I concurred and said that I would be reporting the matter to Higher Authority. I spent most of the evening writing an official report having sought advice regarding the proper procedures from the Adjutant of the LIBTC. After a sleepless night I went to Aldershot in transport provided by the LIBTC and presented my report to the ADDS who was shocked by it and said that he would seek guidance from higher authority about what action should be taken. As I could not work in the Bordon centre again he sent me on leave and I arrived unexpectedly on Heather's doorstep that evening. A few days later I received orders to proceed to Southampton and join the Hospital Ship *Oxfordshire.* This I did in pouring rain on a Sunday afternoon after walking around the docks for some considerable time looking for her. It was several years later that I heard that this particular officer had resigned his commission soon after I left the UK, but had later applied for re-employment during a manpower crisis in the RADC and had his application refused.

The hospital ship *Oxfordshire* was a grand old lady being long in the funnel and four masted. She belonged to the Bibby Line of Liverpool and before the war had been one of their finest ships, sailing regularly between Burma and

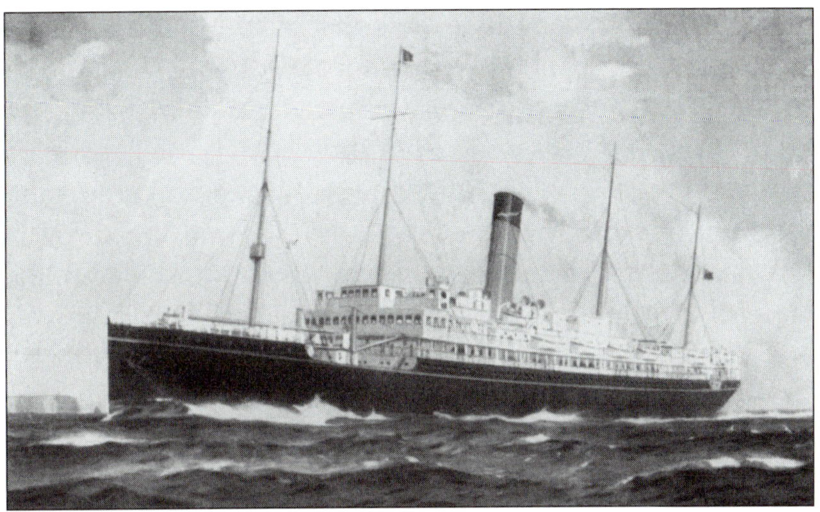

*The Hospital ship* Oxfordshire *in her civilian livery.*

Britain. When I joined her she was an Army ship crewed by British Merchant Navy officers and senior hands, the main crew being Goanese. The medical staff were members of the RAMC, the Nursing Staff were members of the QAIMNS and I, and a Corporal Dental Technician/Dental Clerk Orderly were the sole representatives of the RADC.

I was allocated a cabin on the boat deck which, whilst it had seen better days, still bore signs of its earlier elegance. After stowing my kit I reported to the CO who was attired only in running shorts. I learned later that he was addicted to running round and round the main deck of the ship in an attempt, largely unsuccessful I fear, to lose weight. He was a Lieutenant Colonel who in civilian life had been a Senior Medical Officer in the Prison Medical Service. A mild eccentric he was a charming, amiable man and somewhat surprisingly an excellent CO. He greeted me and suggested that I met my fellow officers in the bar before dinner. This I did and surprised everyone by asking for a soft drink. Little did I know that this was many times more expensive than a double whisky, brandy or gin which cost two and a half old pennies (1p), mixers were also several times more expensive than spirits and beer was sold in litre bottles each costing a pound. Despite my *faux pas* they were a delightful group and we soon became firm friends. They showed me the way down into the officers' dining room which was splendid, the table being laid out formally for a dinner of several courses with white bread rolls neither of which I had seen before, for the wartime National Bread loaf was lightish brown in colour and rationed at that.

The catering on the ship was unbelievable and several choices were available at every meal. We sailed the next morning for an unknown destination. The stokers, who always seem to know these things before the Captain opens his sealed orders, were confident that we were on our way to Japan with whom we were still at war. Their opinions seemed to be confirmed when the first land we saw was Gibraltar as we entered the Mediterranean. The ship was very stable despite some heavy weather and as I had always loved pottering about in boats I loved being at sea.

Quite a few of us were seasick for a couple of days and a certain, unfortunate Corporal Verecchia RAMC was still vomiting and in very poor condition, despite every care when we reached Port Said. He was transferred to a military hospital in Egypt and later flown back to the UK.

We were all allocated to perform various tasks. My first duty was to prepare not only the dental surgery but also the surgical kits that I would need in the Operating Theatre, I was put in charge of the wards on E deck, well below the waterline, and assisted the Nursing Staff to prepare them to receive patients. Later on I was also responsible for the pay and exchange facilities for all patients in the ship as we did not carry any RAPC personnel on board. Time passed quickly. I treated a number of the staff and crew when time and circumstances permitted, read a great deal and whenever possible enjoyed doing this whilst sitting on deck with my back against a lifeboat.

We were all expected to participate fully in the social programme which comprised sing songs, housey housey (bingo), films etc. Our first port of call was Port Said, which has long been known in the British Army as the 'Anus of Creation' and rightly so. We lay at anchor for several days surrounded by 'bum boats' from which black and brown men, who usually claimed to be called Jock McPherson, entreated us to buy a variety of articles including pornographic pictures. When we had a course of enlightening lectures on the horrors of venereal disease the few old soldiers on board knew that we were going to be granted shore leave soon. This we were and as we reached the gangway we were presented with three condoms each, which bore the legend 'Rubber shortage – Is your journey really necessary?' After spending some time in Simon Artz, the famous departmental store in Port Said, we repaired to the officers' club where we had a splendid evening and an excellent meal. I had only just got back to the ship when I had torrential and projectile diarrhoea – the dreaded 'Gyppy Tummy'! I struggled on to my bunk feeling absolutely dreadful and tried unsuccessfully to get to sleep. News of my dilemma spread quickly around the officers' bar and several military and merchant navy officers prepared various concoctions each of which they swore, from personal experience, was the answer to my prayers. They then formed a crocodile at my cabin door each bearing his libation which they administered to me in turn. I knew nothing more until the next morning when I awoke to find that the pain had moved from my abdomen into my head! I later discovered that every one of these concoctions was brandy based, some containing other spirits or liqueurs and some containing unmentionable components. Be that as it may one or other of them had done the trick and I had no more diarrhoea. I realised after this experience, the first time that I had ever drunk alcohol, that drink could have good effects as well as bad ones, so I began to drink alcoholic beverages occasionally.

It was a great surprise to all of us that when we sailed we did not enter the Suez Canal but put out to sea. After some hours we arrived at Haifa in Palestine and entered the harbour and moored alongside a half sunken ship. At hourly intervals an explosion occurred and we were told that these were underwater charges designed to deter frogmen from mining ships berthed in the harbour. Soon after our arrival the light cruiser HMS *Phoebe* berthed alongside a quay in front of us. She looked magnificent as she came in with flags flying at her mast. They were signal flags and the message read 'Oxfordshire. Have you a dentist aboard?' So I was soon treating naval personnel for the first time.

After ridding ourselves of all evidence of identity other than our identity discs and completing the will form in our pay books we were landed by boat and taken to the Carmelite Hospital on Mount Carmel, which was to be our shore base whilst in Haifa. Our duties were to provide medical and dental cover for the area and later to load and evacuate casualties and to assist in the processing of Jewish illegal immigrants. This was a task everyone loathed doing. At the time Jewish refugees were fleeing Europe in their thousands and were being transported in anything that floated, the so-called 'Hell Ships'. Britain had been given a mandate by the League of Nations to govern and maintain law and order in Palestine, a task which became progressively more and more difficult as relationships between Jew and Arab deteriorated. The number of Jewish refugees arriving in Palestinian waters far exceeded the number permitted to settle in the country under international agreements. It became necessary for the Royal Navy and the RAF to institute regular patrols in order that this flow of illegal immigrants be halted. Ships that were intercepted by these patrols were brought into Haifa, the refugees unloaded, put into other vessels and taken to holding camps set up for the purpose in Cyprus. The policy was straightforward but implementing it was a nightmare. Firstly, virtually none of the refugees either spoke or understood English. Secondly, experience had taught them that men in uniform were their enemies and thus to be feared. Fortunately members of my unit did not have to go into the ships and get the people out on to the quay. Those who had this terrible task said that conditions below decks were horrendous and the stench quite sickening. These unfortunates had been packed together like sardines, often lying for days in their own excrement and vomit. Some had died and lay where they had done so. Virtually none of them had experienced either daylight or fresh air from the time that they embarked and all of them were heavily infested. It was our job to disinfect them and to this end a series of canvas screens were set up on the quay behind which this process could be undertaken. At this time no Jewish resident was prepared to assist us and the only Arabs left in the area were converts of the Carmelite monks who, unwanted by Jew or

Arab, were existing in absolute poverty and squalor in the grounds of the monastery on Mount Carmel. As the disinfecting process proceeded, clouds of dust from the powders being used rose above the canvas screens. Quite understandably these pathetic people thought that we were gassing them and so fought us as best they could, kicking, screaming and jumping into the sea in some cases. Somehow the job was done and I realised why the British Tommy has come to be admired for his demeanour and conduct in adversity. When we had dealt with them they were taken out to merchant ships which had been converted to transport them to Cyprus and which had barbed wire barriers around their decks to stop people jumping overboard and so looked anything but inviting.

Britain had announced its intention to give up the mandate and the United Nations was to take over from them. Troops and ships from various countries arrived and proved to be no match for the Stern Gang, the Irgun Zvi Leumi or the Haganah. On the first night that the Americans landed seven of their vehicles were stolen together with arms and ammunition. Meanwhile the British Armed Forces and the Palestine Police Force were withdrawing towards the port of embarkation, Haifa, which was humming with activity as men, vehicles and all forms of equipment were loaded on to ships. Whilst this withdrawal was orderly there were countless incidents and some casualties. We provided medical cover whilst steadily loading the wounded. They were accompanied by the medical staff who had been caring for them and I was joined by Major Bob Harvey, the last RADC officer to serve in the mandate force. A splendid officer and delightful colleague he never stopped working and was an example to everyone. The

*Oxfordshire* was amongst the last ships to leave the harbour on the very last day of the mandate and all on board were pleased to get to sea.

We had an uneventful journey to Port Said where both the casualties and the medical and nursing personnel who had accompanied them were landed. We then set about loading fuel and supplies of all types and made ready to receive casualties when ordered to do so. After a few days these arrived in large numbers, many from the Canal Zone and were of all nationalities. The wards on E deck were allocated to patients in heavy plasters who were unable to take advantage of either exercising or just sitting or lying on the decks. There were also a number of ambulatory patients who were abie to assist in the care of their helpless fellows. Two of the wards were filled with German Afrika Corps casualties whose conduct was admirable. Every bed-bound patient in those wards was fed and watered before the others, all were washed and shaved regularly and their bed spaces were kept immaculate.

After a short stop in Malta we proceeded to Hamburg which together with Harburg and the other nearby communities was absolutely devastated. The channel was lined with sunken or semi sunken ships and rusting hulks and there was an eerie silence as we progressed up the River Elbe. We unloaded our German patients and were given a few days leave in groups and in rotation. This we spent either in the Four Seasons Hotel, an officers' club by the Alster in Hamburg, or in Blankenese, a delightfully fairy tale type of riverside resort which was largely undamaged. We then sailed to Southampton where the remainder of the casualties were landed. After clearing up we were told that the ship was going into reserve and ordered to pack up all the medical equipment. This we did and were sent on leave. As my age and service group was 74 it appeared that my demobilisation was almost due but when it did come up I was one of those deemed Deferred Operationally Vital and not demobilised, due to an acute shortage of dental officers. I was then posted first to Blandford camp in Dorset and then to the Medical Reception Station in Taunton, Somerset and was demobilised a few months later when I joined my uncle's practice as an assistant.

Looking back I realise the value of my military service. One met, lived with and relied upon a variety of people of whose existence I had previously been unaware and I was called upon to deal with situations that I could never have envisaged even in my wildest flights of imagination. It was a maturing experience for me to be a student in the University of Life and I shall always be grateful for it.

It was in the army that I finally lost my faith and became an agnostic. I started having doubts whilst a dental student. The physician under whom I studied medicine was particularly interested in the leukaemias and I spent my days with patients of all ages, some merely babies, afflicted with the disease. In those days the mortality of the disease was for all practical purposes 100%, not like today where it is under 50%. Being young and impressionable I could not comprehend how a God of mercy and a God of love could countenance this and sought guidance from priests of a number of Christian sects all to no avail. The army not only caused me to witness human suffering and misery but also to live in non Christian societies which seemed to me to be composed of a mixture of saints, sinners and in betweens, in similar proportions to Christian societies. In particular I was greatly impressed by the Kibbutz movement, the epitome of socialist Utopia. I started reading comparative theology and philosophy and discovered that virtually all faiths had one central theme summarised by Jesus Christ as 'Love Thy Neighbour'. Whilst I realised that it is much easier to do this and to lead a decent life with the backing of an organised religion I could no longer do this without faith and so was committed to going it alone until I was helped by the Humanist Movement, despite being a non member.

## Chapter Four

# Dental Practice and Medical Studies

I WAS A TOTAL FAILURE in general practice as I was completely hopeless in those business matters which are essential for success. I have never had the slightest interest in money per se and since I joined the army I had had enough to cover my needs which are modest. At the end of a year my uncle was kind enough to offer me a partnership, albeit a very junior one, in the practice. However he was constrained to point out, at some length and giving a number of examples, that I had actually paid those patients that I was most interested in and most enjoyed treating to come rather than making sound economic judgements. I duly reported the offer to Heather that evening saying that I didn't know what to do. Without hesitation she told me that if I accepted the partnership she would be leaving me as the year had been a miserable one, I had been moody and depressed and that it was obvious to her, if not to me, that I was a square peg in a round hole and totally ill equipped to spend the rest of my life in general dental practice. Almost as soon as she stopped speaking, if not before, I knew that she was right. We spent the rest of the evening discussing what I should do and decided that I should look at possible opportunities being created by the introduction of the National Health Service.

I wrote to Clifford Ballard at the Royal telling him of my dilemma and seeking his advice. He invited me to have lunch with him a few days later. When we met he told me that he was setting up postgraduate education in Orthodontics on an in-service basis, that is to say that the students earn their tuition and a small wage by treating hospital patients as they learn. The students would be called stipendiary dental officers and only be paid for the actual hours that they worked on patients. He added that he had only enough funding to pay two or three stipendiaries for two and a half days a week. He told me of his belief that proper postgraduate training in the dental specialities, which had been virtually non existent before the war, was bound to come as it already had in Oral Surgery in the armed forces. He reminded me that the Royal College of Surgeons of England had set up a Faculty of Dental Surgery and a Fellowship by examination. When I told Heather what he had said she was enthusiastic although it appeared that I would have to continue to work part time in practice to make ends meet. I therefore applied for the programme and was accepted. When I arrived back at the Royal I was very pleasantly surprised to be offered a similar opportunity to train in Oral Surgery for the other half of the week. This I accepted although I realised that I would have to go back to working evenings, weekends etc. in practice to keep my head above water. I thoroughly enjoyed the next few months for Clifford had been joined by John Hovell, an ex-army consultant in both Orthodontics and Oral Surgery, and John Hooper, a dentally qualified ex prisoner of war, who later had the distinction of being appointed as the first Regional Consultant Orthodontist in the National Health Service.

They were all gifted clinicians and great enthusiasts and co-operated splendidly to create a most lively and stimulating environment. The Oral Surgery programme suffered from a multiplicity of part time consultants no two of whom had similar views, although a number of them were impressive clinicians. I was struck by the different approach to practice of the medically and dentally qualified consultants when compared to those who were dentally qualified alone and decided, after taking advice from some of them, to apply for admission to the Middlesex Hospital Medical School. This I did and was granted an interview with its distinguished Dean, Sir Harold Boldero. All but one of the four dental consultants at the Middlesex were Royal trained and two of them were also consultants there. Both institutions had had strong links in the past and so he was sympathetic to my cause. However a difficulty arose because I had not taken the 1st MB Examination of London University but the Pre Medical Examination of the Royal Colleges, for during the war university examinations in dentistry had been suspended. Middlesex, like all the medical schools in London was only running university degree courses which were one year longer than diploma courses. Sir Harold said that he would accept me as a student and sign me up for the LRCP (London) MRCS (Eng) examinations if I would agree to doing the full degree course, and did not ask for any exemptions or special treatment. I was happy to do this for although it would delay my qualification in medicine by one year it would provide me with greater opportunities to earn some money in practice, for I knew that I had to work my passage.

I entered Medical School in October 1949 having resigned my Oral Surgery post at the Royal and, by agreement with Clifford, reduced the number of my sessions in Orthodontics. My year in medical school consisted largely of other ex servicemen with relatively few school leavers. Thus they were a worldly and a lively group of medical students who were determined to take full advantage of the great opportunity afforded them to build a new life for themselves. A number of them later had distinguished careers in a wide range of medical disciplines. At that time the Middlesex Hospital Medical School was fortunate enough to have a most able and distinguished staff, Professors Samson Wright and Slome in Physiology, Professors Kirk, Walls and Silver in Anatomy, Professor Sir Charles Dodds and Drs Holt and Jepson in Biochemistry, and many others who saw the potential of such students and capitalised on it by creating an exciting academic environment for them which I for one thoroughly enjoyed. Such was the standard of teaching in Basic Medical Sciences at the Middlesex that after taking the 2nd examination of the Conjoint Board upon completing the course I was fortunate enough to be awarded the Begley Prize of the Royal College of Surgeons of England, in March 1951, an unexpected honour which raised my stock in the Medical School and my bank balance a trifle. It also gave me the confidence to take the Primary Dental Fellowship Examinations a few weeks later which I managed to pass without undue difficulty.

This was the time when the newspapers were sensationalising the high incomes being earned by NHS dentists working excessive hours to cope with the rush of patients able to obtain proper dental treatment for the first time, and I am sure that many of my teachers and fellow students wondered what I was doing as an impecunious medical student. Although I only had seventeen pounds in the world when I joined the medical school my wife had steadily advanced in her Civil Service posts in the Air Ministry and there was plenty of part time out of hours work available in NHS general practice so we were able to rent a small flat in a terraced house and enjoy our lives together. We joined the Little Ship Club and attended courses in seamanship and navigation at Beaver Hall on Garlick Hill in the City each week in the winter and crewed in other people's boats during the sailing season. We were regular members of the crew of an old clinker built 35ft ketch named *Redskin* which was berthed in Heybridge Basin near Maldon, Essex and spent many happy weekends working on her and sailing in Essex and Suffolk waters. One summer we agreed to spend our holidays sailing on the Dutch Waterways in the company of the owner and his wife and another amateur crew member. We set out from Harwich for Ijmuiden at the mouth of the North Sea Canal which goes to Amsterdam. Unfortunately we were caught up in the worst gale experienced in the North Sea for decades and lost both our storm trisail and the two sea anchors which we constructed as well as a hatch cover. The motion of the boat was unbelievable and could only be compared to being in a lift gone mad. One minute one was on the crest of a wave and could see for miles the next we were at the bottom of a trough and the tips of the waves appeared to be mast high. Everyone but me was seasick although the skipper, fortunately, was not as ill as the others. Heather was terribly sick and I had to lash her in to stop her going overboard. He was able to keep the engine running whilst I struggled to keep her bows into the wind. After many hours the wind dropped to a level where it was safe to approach land and we found a buoy which we identified as being off Zeebruge in Belgium. As we entered the harbour we were surprised to find the cones still hoisted indicating that the wind was still of gale force and to be told by the customs man who came aboard that no fishing vessel had gone to sea for three or four days, and that two yachts had foundered, only then did we realise how lucky we had been. To this day I do not understand why I was not seasick on that occasion as I have been in much milder conditions. The others could not wait to go ashore but I did not bother to do so and occupied myself on the boat drying out and effecting repairs with the help of the locals. We sailed up the Dutch coast stopping at Middleburg and Scheveningen and entered the canal system at Ijmuiden as originally planned, albeit over a week late. We spent the next three weeks exploring the canals and traversing the Ijsselmeer (formerly the Zuider Zee) and went down to Rotterdam. We had an idyllic time and were overwhelmed by the friendliness and hospitality of the Dutch who could not have been kinder or more hospitable. We had an uneventful passage home from the Hook of Holland to Harwich and on to Heybridge Basin but that was the end of sailing for Heather for many years.

Like all other ex servicemen of my generation I was an army reservist and so fully expected to be recalled to the colours at the time of the Berlin Air Lift crisis. In the event I was not but the Cold War made it possible that I would be sometime. I decided that if I had to go I would prefer to go as a member of a unit rather than as an individual and so sought a suitable vacancy in the Territorial Army. At that time there were only about a dozen or so posts for RADC officers mainly on the establishments of TA General Hospitals, most of which were already filled. I was fortunate enough to hear of a vacancy in the 17th (London) General Hospital RAMC (TA) based at the Duke of York's Headquarters in Chelsea. After being interviewed by its

Commanding Officer, Colonel Mitchell Heggs, who in civilian life was a distinguished Consultant Dermatologist at St Mary's Hospital, Paddington, my application for it was accepted and my long association with the TA and TAVR began. More of that later because it was important enough in my life to warrant a chapter of its own. However it had one side effect worthy of mention here in that the monies I received in pay and annual bounties from the TA enabled Heather and me to spend our annual holidays cruising as passengers in cargo ships to Norway, Denmark, Holland, Germany and both French and Spanish Morocco all of which we thoroughly enjoyed.

There was a wonderful spirit in the Middlesex Hospital which was carefully nurtured by the staff. Great emphasis was laid on the fact that the patients were the most important people in the institution, our *raison d'être*, and that they were not interesting cases but fellow human beings with a problem. The standard of nursing care was superb and all medical students spent one month doing the same duties on the wards as probationer nurses at the commencement of their clinical studies. A revealing and rewarding sojourn on bed pan alley! This was a period of great change in medicine as drug and vaccine therapy brought the infectious diseases, including such killers as tuberculosis and poliomyelitis, under control and advances in anaesthesia made lung and heart surgery possible. Advances were being made in every branch of medicine and surgery and it was a very exciting time to be a medical student. There were also many extra curricular activities to participate in both formal and informal. As in dental school I won colours in football and once again failed to get into either the University or United Hospitals teams. I was Honorary Secretary of several

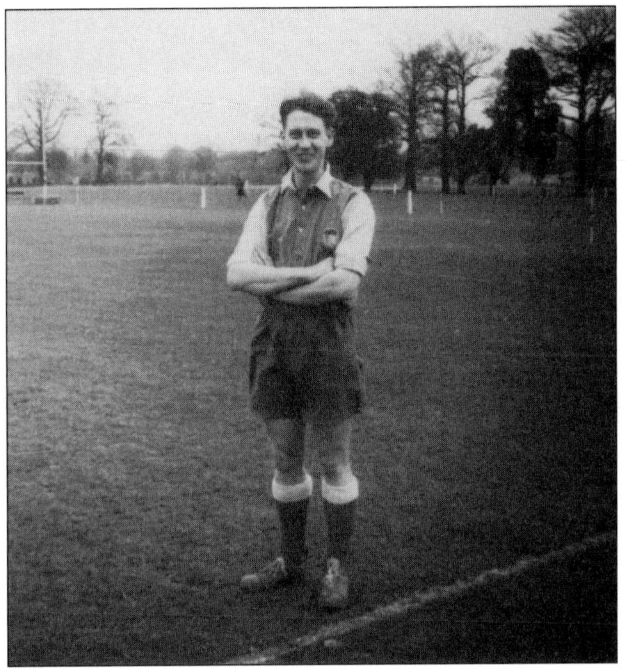

*As a member of Middlesex Hospital AFC.*

student societies and of the Annual Smoking Concert held at the Scala Theatre at which such artists as Tommy Cooper, Sam Costa, Brian Rix etc. gave their services free in Aid of Cancer Research. Whenever a staff shortage occurred in the Dental Department of the Middlesex I used to be asked by the consultants from the Royal who ran it to lend a hand and did so often deputising for the Resident Dental Officer. In October 1951 I was appointed a part time clinical assistant in the Dental Department and resigned my stipendiary post at the Royal. The duties were mainly in oral surgery on both in and out patients but I also attended the weekly Head and Neck Cancer Clinic run by Professor Sir Brian Windeyer, an outstanding radiotherapist and Mr C.P. Wilson, one of the most talented Head and Neck oncologists of his day. Both always treated me with great courtesy and valued my dental expertise and the contributions that I made both to discussions leading to the formulation of treatment plans and during actual treatment. Never once did they allude to the unusual fact that I was only a medical student. I held the Clinical Assistant post until I qualified in medicine in January 1954.

By this time legislation had been introduced which required new medical graduates to hold two recognised house appointments before becoming fully registered medical practitioners. Competition for such posts was intense, especially in teaching hospitals, and so, in common with my fellow graduates, I applied for all such posts available at the Middlesex. There followed a fortnight of interviews, tests etc. as individual consultants drew up their lists in order of preference each using his or her own criteria. There was then a Special Meeting of the Medical Committee at which the individual appointments were decided, the most Senior Physician having the first choice and the most Senior Surgeon the second and so on in order of seniority. Whilst this process was going on all the applicants were required to gather in the Front Hall of the Hospital and await the results. I can still remember the tense atmosphere and the shock that I got when it was announced that I was appointed to be House Physician to Dr D. Evan Bedford and Dr Walter Somerville in the Cardiology Department. My surprise was not only because I had never been a student on their firm and had never shown the slightest interest in being a physician in general or a cardiologist in particular but Dr Evan Bedford was a clinician of world repute, the Senior Physician of the Hospital and known to be extremely difficult to serve. One of my fellow graduates who happened to have the same surname as I, was extremely interested in Cardiology and well qualified for the post and so I asked if an error had been made, the first of my many mistakes whilst working on the Firm, for it was immediately pointed out to me that God, in the form of Dr Bedford, did not make such mistakes!

During the next six months I soon came to recognise how fortunate I had been for both my chiefs and their Senior Registrar, Dr Richard Emmanuel, were all superb clinicians and excellent teachers. For years Dr Bedford and his team had meticulously recorded details of their patient's medical histories and related their findings during extensive clinical examinations, especially of abnormal heart sounds heard during auscultation to post-mortem findings. Thus when Sir Thomas Holme Sellors began to perform heart surgery at the Middlesex they were able to tell him the precise nature of the valvular lesions of each patient presenting for surgery, and so assist him in the selection of those patients most likely to benefit from procedures such as mitral valvotomy. They also provided intensive medical treatment prior to surgery thus ensuring that such patients were in optimum condition when they went to the operating theatre and undertook their post operative care, thus giving them the maximum chance of recovery. In this they were supported by a devoted and specialised nursing team led by a remarkable woman, Miriam Hammond, who had been the Sister in Charge of the Cardiology Unit for two decades and was the only person I knew who could wind Dr Bedford around her little finger. The results of this teamwork were spectacular and amongst the best anywhere in the world.

I found myself responsible for the day to day care of thirty very ill patients, many of whom had either coronary artery disease or severe hypertension or both. New drugs, including hypotensives, which lower the blood pressure, were being introduced and experience was being gained in their use and unwanted side effects. I learned the importance of patience and encouragement during history taking, for many patients have difficulty in describing their symptoms and lack the knowledge of what is important and what is unimportant. I was taught the value of thorough and meticulous clinical examination as a routine and soon came to appreciate the benefits of good nursing. I learned much from my senior colleagues but even more from Sister Hammond who seemed to always appear as my mentor and guide at critical moments. I worked enormously long hours for, in addition to taking my turn as first doctor on call in the Casualty Department at nights and weekends, I was also responsible for all electrocardiograms required everywhere in the hospital out of hours.

Patients who had suffered heart attacks were often admitted as emergencies at night and also everyone knew that I was dentally qualified and so called upon my expertise when patients presented with facial injuries or dental emergencies. At this time Heather had an important and demanding job at the Air Ministry and so we only had one meal a week together during which I often went to sleep. Fortunately she was very understanding and supportive despite being very concerned for my health and welfare. I matured rapidly in this job. On my very first night as a House Physician I was called to the ward at two o'clock in the morning to see a male patient with severe respiratory difficulties and conducted a clinical examination on a bright blue man coughing and spluttering and fighting for his breath. With some difficulty I found that he had a large pleural effusion and that one lung had collapsed. I decided to drain the effusion with the assistance of the Night Sister. I had just inserted the needle and drained off a copious amount of blood stained fluid when the patient rolled off the needle dead. Our efforts at resuscitation failed and we retired to the ward kitchen and made ourselves some tea, over which we discussed what had happened and reviewed what we had done, and discussed whether we should have proceeded differently or done anything more. This discussion was interrupted regularly as Night Sister did her rounds leaving me alone with my thoughts. I was still there when Richard Emmanuel arrived early the next morning. He told me that the patient had been terminally ill with widespread cancer and severe heart disease for several weeks, and that my clinical decisions had been correct although no one could have saved the patient. After a post-mortem had confirmed his statements he immediately sent for me and told me, adding that all young doctors had to learn that they were not God!

When the hypotensive drugs were introduced it was hoped that another major medical problem had been solved. Since then there have been great developments in the field and enormous progress has been made, although some problems still await solution. When I was a house physician we were still 'feeling our way' with the first hypotensives to be introduced. A male patient was admitted in severe congestive heart failure and to my horror I found that his blood pressure was too high to be recorded on a sphygmomanometer. He was put on a salt free diet, which is singularly unappetising and given diuretics and hypotensives in gradually increasing doses. His physical condition improved dramatically and we were delighted until we discovered that as his blood pressure approached normal limits his mental state deteriorated and a delightful cultured person became a zombie. Recognising that this was probably due to a diminished blood supply to the brain when his high blood pressure was controlled, we spent the next two months trying to find a happy medium in which his blood pressure was reduced enough to allow his heart failure to be controlled. We failed to do so and a clinical conference was held at which it was decided to stop the treatment and allow him to have whatever food and drink he wanted and spend his last few weeks living as a real person rather than existing as a 'cabbage'. As I had to implement this decision on a day to day basis I was grateful to my senior colleagues who reminded me that the great Arab physician of antiquity, Avicena, had written that the treatment should never be worse than the disease and that it had long been held that 'Thou shalt not kill, but shall not strive officiously to keep alive'.

This patient had not been in any position to influence the decision but most patients and or their families are, and their decisions can cause problems of implementation. I admitted a lovely 28 year old mother of two in congestive heart failure due to rheumatic valvular heart disease. Against all advice she had become pregnant again and it soon became apparent that it was going to be more and more difficult to control her heart failure as her pregnancy progressed. Although her valvular lesion was far from ideal for surgery Sir Thomas managed to perform a successful mitral valvotomy and her condition improved. Unfortunately this improvement was not maintained and it became obvious that only a termination of pregnancy could save her life, and I was deputed to explain this to both the patient and her husband who were known to be staunch Roman Catholics. After several discussions and much soul searching they consented to the operation and signed the necessary forms, greatly to my relief, and arrangements were made for surgery the next day. The next morning I was called to the ward to be told that following a visit to the ward by the Hospital's Roman Catholic chaplain, consent to the operation had been withdrawn. After discussions with both the patient and her husband I had no alternative but to accept their decision although it condemned me to caring for her every day until she died nearly three months later, despite our best efforts. I liked the Roman Catholic Chaplain as a man and respected his integrity but was never able to bring myself to talk to him again.

As the reader will have gathered this first house post was an important milestone in my career and I could relate many other anecdotes about it, some serious and some, such as Dr Bedford's eccentricities, humorous. Suffice it to say that for the first time in my life I realised that I could have enjoyed being a physician and I have always been grateful for the lessons that I learned as a very junior member of a splendid unit.

Relatively few of my contemporaries obtained a second house appointment at the Middlesex and so I counted myself extremely fortunate to be appointed as ENT house surgeon. My chiefs were Messrs C.P. Wilson, J.P. Monkhouse and Sir Douglas Ranger. The latter two were particularly interested in deafness and developing surgical techniques to alleviate certain forms of it and I greatly enjoyed assisting them. However most of my time was spent working with 'C.P.' once again. He was a head and neck surgeon and his main interest was the treatment of cancer.

He had been an anatomist for sixteen years and was a superb dissector and an imaginative and courageous surgeon. Many of his patients had undergone radiotherapy treatment some time before coming under his care and so their tissues were distorted by scarring and to see him dissect out and display vital structures whilst dealing with malignancies was both a privilege and a delight. His surgical judgement and tissue craft were outstanding and ensured that the results of his surgery were the envy of most of his peers. His skills salvaged the lives of many patients thought to be untreatable by others. As a person he could be extremely difficult to work with and was a very hard task master. Fortunately I had earned his respect when working with him as a clinical assistant and he took great pains to help me develop practical surgical skills even allowing me to perform major operations such as removal of the voice box (laryngectomy) and removal of the upper jaw (maxillectomy), under his guidance as he acted as my assistant during these surgical procedures towards the end of my appointment.

At the end of six months he invited Heather and me to have dinner with him during which he suggested that I trained as a head and neck surgeon under his guidance rather than completing my training as an oral surgeon as I had planned. At that time I had passed the Primary Dental Fellowship but had not attempted the Primary Surgical Fellowship. He suggested that I spent the next few months preparing for this examination and knowing that I was impecunious generously offered to support me financially whilst I did this. Both Heather and I were astounded at his kindness and generosity and agreed to consider his offer seriously. This we did and during the next few days Heather got me to detail in writing the various stages in training that

I would have to undertake to obtain consultant status in each of the two specialities together with an approximate time scale for each. When these were confirmed it became obvious that acceptance of 'C.P.'s' offer would entail one or two more years in training than sticking to our original plans. Although much of this time would be 'in service' the relevant training posts were few and far between, had to be obtained in open competition with other candidates and were poorly paid. Heather expressed her concern that I was in danger of becoming a perpetual student to the exclusion of family life and so we decided to stick to our original plan. 'C.P.' was extremely gracious and understanding when I told him of our decision and expressed the hope that I would apply for a consultant post at the Middlesex when qualified to do so.

The next two or three months were anxious ones for I needed a registrar post in Oral Surgery and no vacancies were advertised. In order to earn a living I obtained any locum work that I could find often being a medical practitioner for a part of the day and a dental surgeon for the rest of it. A friend of mine was the Medical Superintendent of the Shaw, Saville and Albion Line and in this capacity was going on the maiden voyage of their fine new liner, the *Southern Cross*, to Australia. Knowing that I was doubly qualified he invited me to accompany him as his assistant. I was sorely tempted to do so but in the next issue of the *British Dental Journal* not one, but three vacancies for Registrars in Oral Surgery were advertised and so I applied for all three. Having read the details of the posts I considered that the one at the Eastman Dental Hospital (Postgraduate Institute of the University of London) was the most desirable of the three and so was both delighted and relieved to be shortlisted for interview for that post first. I was surprised to be the only candidate called for interview and my surprise was compounded when immediately after the interview I was offered the job on the spot and told that as it was vacant I could start work on the following Monday morning. I was overjoyed to find that I would be working for Sir William Kelsey Fry and the Dean of the Institute, Professor Frank Wilkinson, two major figures in the speciality, and accepted the post immediately. That night I treated Heather to a celebratory scallop and lobster dinner, our favourite, at Manzi's famous fish restaurant just off Leicester Square.

## Chapter Five

# In Service Training

DURING THE First World War a young ENT surgeon, Captain Harold Gillies, was posted to the Cambridge Military Hospital in Aldershot with orders to set up a unit to treat patients who had sustained facial injuries. Prior to this the treatment of such war wounded soldiers had left much to be desired and was completely ad hoc. Gillies, an unorthodox New Zealander, was soon deluged with patients transferred from other military hospitals in which they had been vegetating and set about his mammoth task with his characteristic enthusiasm and flair. He soon realised that he needed dental assistance and went to the CO of the hospital asking for it. At that time the Army Dental Corps did not exist and there were only a handful of dental surgeons serving as officers on the General List. The CO told him that none of these were available and suggested that he went up to the Officers Ward where there was a dentally qualified patient, with whom he could discuss his problems. This patient was Captain William Kelsey Fry who had been wounded in action whilst serving as a Regimental Medical Officer in the front line. This chance encounter was to lead to the development of the specialities of plastic surgery and oral and maxillofacial surgery in the United Kingdom, for as soon as he was fit enough to do so Kelsey Fry spent his convalescence working with Gillies, a partnership which was to last until the Second World War broke out. Between the two wars they worked together in the country's only Plastic and Oral Surgery Centre which was housed in a Ministry of Pensions hospital, St Mary's Hospital, Sidcup, albeit on a part time basis, for Gillies was a Consultant at Barts whilst Kelsey Fry was on the staff of Guy's.

In 1938 they were charged with the task of setting up a series of Maxillofacial Centres throughout the country as war was thought to be imminent. This they did and Gillies chose to head the Unit at Rooksdown House, Basingstoke, whilst Kelsey Fry chose to go to the Queen Victoria Hospital, East Grinstead. Sir William told me that Sir Harold chose Rooksdown House because of the excellent fly fishing there, whilst his choice was governed by the proximity of the boarding school that his son attended! At the Cambridge Military Hospital they were joined by a surgeon named Henry Tonks who was also a distinguished artist who later became Master of the Slade School. Clinical photography had not been developed in those days and so Tonks recorded their cases in a series of drawings. These priceless records are housed in the Royal College of Surgeons of England and Kelsey Fry used to encourage his juniors, including me, to look at and learn from them. Many years later whilst serving on the Council of the Royal College I learned that the drawings had been put into storage as there was no space available to display them. At the time I was a trustee of the Royal Army Dental Corps museum which had just been opened at the Corps depot in Aldershot and was able to arrange for the drawings to be displayed there.

Sir William was in his sixties when I worked for him and was by then an established and well respected figure in World Dentistry. He was an accomplished prosthetist and

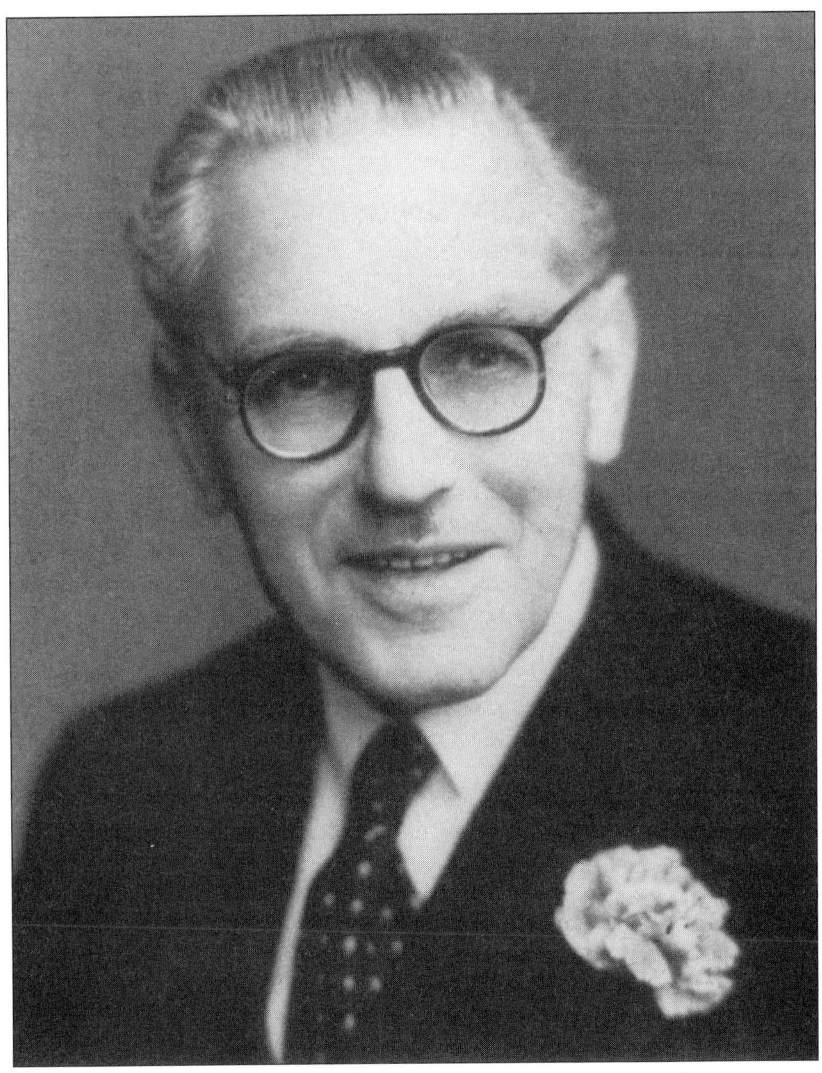

*Sir William Kelsey Fry, my mentor and role model.*

headed the Prosthetic Department at Guy's for many years. A brilliant diagnostician, a careful if rather conservative surgeon and a born teacher who believed in learning by experience and teaching by example, he was invariably courteous and correct in dealing with everyone, a gentleman of the old school. He had a wonderful clinical memory and could remember details of many patients under his care decades earlier, when their condition was relevant to the care of another patient. He possessed an enquiring mind and constantly urged his juniors to ask themselves whether they could have done things better or differently to the benefit of the patient. He was constantly asking probing questions the commonest of which was 'Why?' I admired him greatly and he rapidly became my role model.

Professor Frank Wilkinson was cast in an entirely different mould. The son of a Mersey pilot he was proud of his northern roots. He gave up a lucrative private practice in Rodney Street in Liverpool to become Dean of the ailing dental school in Melbourne, Australia. Under his guidance it became the finest dental school in the Antipodes and he was invited to become Dean of the Dental School in the Victoria University of Manchester. He was an outstanding success in this post and persuaded an industrialist, Sir Samuel Turner, to finance the rebuilding of the Dental School. The Eastman had never been a success as a Postgraduate Institute despite being staffed by young enthusiastic up and coming specialists in all the dental disciplines. It was said that there were too many prima donnas singing solos and too few team members singing together. Be that as it may, Professor Wilkinson was invited to become the Dean and, after telling some staff members their fortunes in his traditional blunt northern way and banging a few heads together, soon turned the tide. Ably assisted by Sir William, Clifford Ballard, Ivor Kramer, John Lee, Dick Stephens, George Cross, Guy Morrant et al, he ushered in a Golden Age in the Eastman and made it the place that almost everyone with any ambition in dentistry wanted to be part of. He made his top priority the improvement of clinical standards in dental practice and to this end instituted regular postgraduate refresher courses for general dental practitioners in every dental discipline. The newly instituted dental fellowship (FDS RCS Eng) had quickly become the postgraduate diploma to obtain and the Royal College had instituted excellent revision courses in the basic medical sciences for candidates preparing to sit the Primary Fellowship examination. Great teachers who participated in these courses included an Australian anatomist, Professor Last, Professor Slome, my teacher in Physiology at the Middlesex and Drs John Walters and Alan Reese, fellow officers of mine in 17th (London) General Hospital RAMC (TA), both of whom had coached me in Pathology and especially Morbid Histology whilst I was a medical student. Professor Wilkinson set up a three month long full time course for candidates preparing for the Final Fellowship examination to complement this Primary course. Such were the examination successes of those who had taken this course that the Eastman was besieged with potential students from all over the country and indeed the world and especially from all corners of the Commonwealth. As Clifford Ballard had made his department the place to be in orthodontics the Eastman was full of enthusiastic, bright and able young dentists keen to learn and exchange ideas. The atmosphere was electric and I learned much over coffee and the lunch table. Prior to this time dental schools had been rather insular and introspective and learning what people from other schools in this and other countries had been taught to do and believe in was a salutary experience for all of us.

On arrival at the Eastman to take up my post I was met by a rather harassed colleague, Dr R. Gordon Mitchell, who was Senior Registrar on Sir William's firm at the time. He told me that due to sickness amongst the staff he and I were the only staff on duty to cope with a large number of patients with dental emergencies, supervise Fellowship students removing impacted wisdom teeth under local anaesthesia and prepare for a general practitioner course due to start on Thursday. Thus began a lifelong friendship with the future first Dental Superintendent of the new Birmingham Dental Hospital. Gordon was a New Zealander who had qualified in both medicine and dentistry in Manchester when Professor Wilkinson was Dean there. A quiet man he was particularly interested in what is now known as Oral Medicine especially actinomycosis and facial pain. This latter interest was also shared with Sir William to whom Gordon was devoted. Sir William thought the world of him and admired the way that he ran the surgical component of the FDS course on a day to day basis, despite never having sat for the Primary examination. This was no mean feat for David Downton who was First Assistant on Professor Wilkinson's firm was not medically qualified but had the Fellowship. He was a gifted operator who espoused practice rather than theory. Thus they were not always facing the same way on the tandem that circumstances forced them to ride. It was obvious to me that I had come into a hothouse and that I was going to have to tread carefully and work extremely hard if I was going to make the grade.

I decided to make completion of the Fellowship

examination my first objective and whenever time and circumstances permitted I attended those parts of the FDS course which dealt with my deficiencies in knowledge. The lectures on Oral Pathology given by Ivor Kramer, who had been a student about three years senior to me at the Royal, were particularly outstanding not only in content but in presentation. As I knew Ivor to be a rather shy and introverted backroom boy I realised how much thought and planning had gone into each presentation. I picked his brains quite ruthlessly in an endeavour to improve my teaching techniques. In a few months I passed the final FDS examination, Sir William, an examiner being one of the first to congratulate me upon my success. He went on to express his concern that due to personal circumstances and pressure of work Gordon had never attempted the Fellowship examinations. He asked me if I would take on some of Gordon's duties in order to give him a chance to remedy this deficiency. I readily agreed to do so and was privileged to run Sir William's Outpatient Consultant Clinics and Inpatient Operating sessions, being given more and more responsibility as the months went by. Sir William was a most able clinician and an inspiring and stimulating teacher who could always be relied upon to introduce a new facet when discussing even the most mundane of cases. His clinics were a magnet for distinguished colleagues from elsewhere and were often followed by intriguing discussions over a meal. Like Gordon I soon became devoted to him and began to share some of his special interests, in my case the management of facial pain and the rehabilitation of denture cripples. The latter are a group of unfortunates who become estranged from their fellows because of their inability to wear dentures following the loss of their natural dentition, making it difficult for them to converse or enjoy their meals in company. Gordon passed both parts of the Fellowship at his first attempt and returned to full duty.

It was arranged for me to spend some time each week in the Prosthetic Department under the guidance of John Lee and Alan Lawson in order to study the problem in depth from a prosthetic point of view. It was a revelation to me to find prosthetics being practised on a biological basis rather than a mechanical one and to see surgery being employed to deal with anatomical obstacles to prosthetic success. These surgical techniques were being developed by David Downton who at that time had more experience in tuberosity reduction and mylohyoid ridge resection than anyone else. He had extremely good surgical hands and his superb handling of old atrophied and friable soft tissues was both a joy to behold and the basis of his success in this difficult and demanding field. He was kind enough to take me under his wing and to teach me all he knew and the subject became my main research interest and absorbed my attention for many years as I tried to evolve a series of plastic surgery procedures within the mouth to deal with various anatomical obstacles to prosthetic success. The months passed quickly as I honed both my clinical and teaching skills in this ideal environment and I matured as a clinician. However I had not worked in a regional maxillofacial unit since my student house surgeon days and lacked experience in the management of trauma. Thus with the encouragement of both Sir William and Professor Wilkinson I answered an advertisement for a Senior Registrar post in Oral Surgery in the Welsh Regional Plastic and Oral Surgery Centre then based at St Lawrence's Hospital at Chepstow in Monmouthshire, and was fortunate enough to be appointed, and to enter yet another different world.

St Lawrence's was a wartime hospital housed in a series of wooden huts and had orthopaedic and chest units in addition to the plastic and oral surgery units which were required to treat all the maxillofacial injuries and burns sustained by patients in Mid and South Wales. To this end the staff, including me, the only Senior Registrar in Oral Surgery in Wales, were required to travel, hold clinics and operate in a series of other hospitals. The workload was immense and the surgical teams small so I was required to be resident in the hospital. In my experience many plastic surgeons seem to be small in stature and suffer from the little Napoleon complex. Emlyn Lewis was in this mould and extremely difficult to work with. He was however an immensely experienced and outstandingly competent surgeon who took an especial interest in me and from whom I learned much. The oral surgery consultant in the unit was a delightful Bristol graduate named John Gibson who whilst not being medically qualified was vastly experienced and extremely competent. He was quiet and shy by nature, sensitive and self effacing. Not surprisingly he did not greatly enjoy working with Emlyn Lewis and preferred working with the other plastic surgeons, Len Scofield and Mike Tempest, in a more relaxed fashion. He was a joy to work for and although he would be the first to deny it taught me many things. The Chief Anaesthetist on the unit was a jovial Irishman named Larry Middleton who in addition to being a master of his craft coped well with Emlyn Lewis and his tantrums. He went on to win a National award for his skills. I was extremely grateful for his presence and support during the frequent prolonged nocturnal emergency operations when I was acting as surgical assistant to my plastic surgery chief.

Every Wednesday I got up at the crack of dawn and drove to Morriston Hospital in Swansea. In those days the roads were bad and so the journey took a couple of hours or even longer if there was a hold up at the level crossing in the middle of Port Talbot. My chief in Swansea was Tom Richards who was very Welsh and had a roguish sense of humour and a constant twinkle in his eye. He was a dental consultant of the old school who made no secret of the fact that he had never had any formal training in oral surgery. We got on well and he trusted my surgical judgement and was kind enough to say that he envied me my surgical skills. Our working day commenced with a Consultants Clinic which was followed by an inpatient operating session under general anaesthesia during which he was always prepared to act as my surgical assistant. After lunch, which was often a late lunch, I drove back to the Neath General Hospital where I did another operating list under general anaesthesia on my own.

The contrast between the two hospitals was striking. Morriston had been an EMS hospital and was set in the most beautiful grounds inhabited by peacocks. It had developed into the major hospital facility in West Wales and had an outstanding Medical Superintendent and a large well qualified Consultant staff. In contrast Neath General was run down and poorly equipped. Nevertheless I enjoyed working there, largely because my anaesthetist, John Davies, was a splendid fellow and extremely competent. He was singularly responsible for the maintenance of high standards of patient care in that hospital to which he was devoted. He had never had the opportunity to obtain the Fellowship in

Anaesthesia and so did not enjoy consultant status. We became firm friends and I realised that his problem would be to prepare for the basic sciences examinations in the Primary due to his isolation from an academic centre and crippling workload. Together we devised a study plan to overcome this problem and I persuaded him to obtain a few weeks study leave and enrol on the revision course held at the Royal College of Surgeons in London. This he did and waltzed through both the Primary and Final examinations in rapid succession. All his colleagues and admirers were delighted when he obtained his consultant status in the hospital that he both graced and served so well throughout his life. We often did not finish the operating list until early evening and I then drove back to Chepstow, tired but well satisfied with my day's work only to find an emergency admission or two awaiting my return. Tom Richards introduced me to the Mumbles and the Gower Peninsula which I came to love very much, and still do.

After I had been enjoying myself at Chepstow for almost a year John Gibson came into my surgery one morning and asked me if I had seen a copy of the current British Dental Journal. When I replied in the negative he told me that there was an advertisement in it for a Senior Registrar in Oral Surgery at the Eastman, the wording of which could roughly be translated as a call for me to return. I told him that I was enjoying working with him and learning a great deal and did not want to leave. He was kind enough to say that he did not want to lose me but as consultant jobs were few and far between my chances of obtaining one in a couple of years time would be enhanced if I was coming from the Eastman with the backing of Sir William and Professor Wilkinson rather than from Chepstow with his backing. After a restless night I decided not to apply and told John so. He queried the wisdom of my decision but admitted that personally he was delighted by it. Some weeks passed by and I received a letter saying that I had been shortlisted for the post and summoning me to attend for interview. John insisted that I did so saying that it would be discourteous to say the least to snub two chiefs who had been so kind as to take an interest in me. Once again I was the only candidate interviewed and was offered the job and pressed to take it. Heather was still living in our flat in Tooting and so I promised to give my answer after discussing the matter with her. When I did so I got a good telling off for not listening to John's wise counsel and risking offending two of the key figures in my professional life.

Thus I returned to the Eastman and soon found out why I had been pressured into returning for Gordon Mitchell had left to take up his Consultancy in Birmingham, and Professor Wilkinson had departed on a visit to the Antipodes whilst Sir William went to America for a month or two leaving me to 'hold the fort' in the department. This I did with the assistance of such excellent registrars as Lester Kay, Eric Morgan, Maurice Jones, Patrick James etc. in the succeeding months. The department settled down into a smooth running routine, our examination successes continued and one had time to indulge in research activity and contribute papers to learned journals.

Like Professor Wilkinson many of us were keen on sailing. He was reputed to have won an Around Tasmania race with a crew of dental students whilst Dean of the Melbourne School, and was a most accomplished yachtsman. Each summer we chartered a yacht and set off, often from Dartmouth, for a fortnight's sailing usually

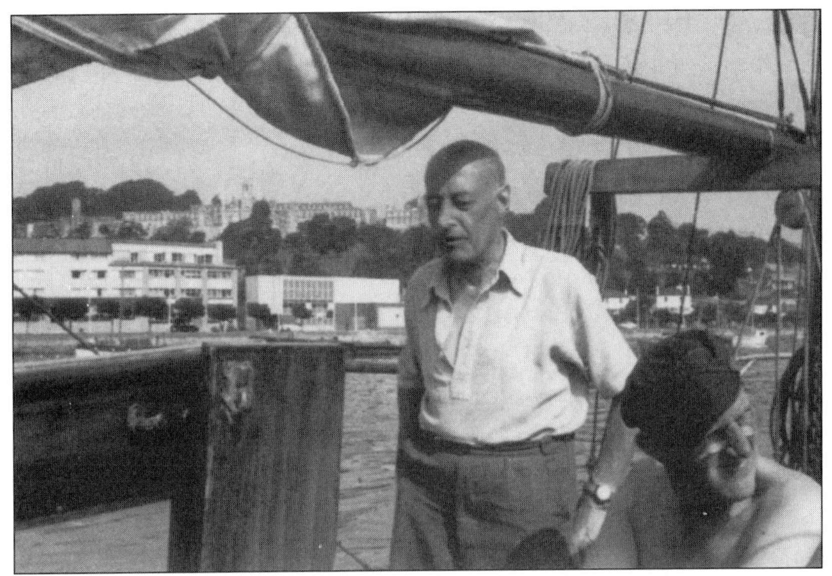

*In harbour. 'Prof' Wilkinson and Patrick James.*

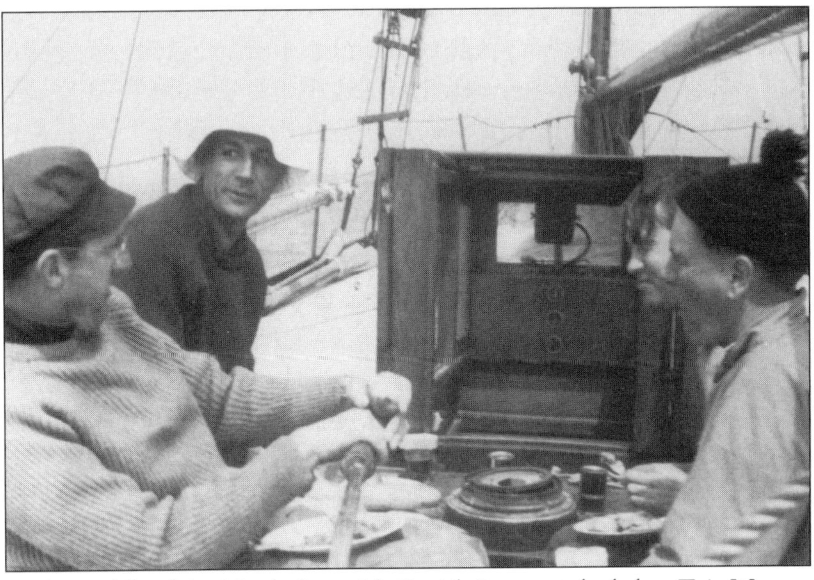

*In the middle of the North Sea with Patrick James at the helm, Eric Morgan in the floppy hat and a tasselled Ray O'Neil.*

around Brittany and the Channel Islands with the Professor as skipper. We repeated this practice for a number of years and were joined by other colleagues such as Rupert Sutton Taylor, a consultant at the Westminster Hospital and Ray O'Neil, then a consultant at Guy's, who became Professor of Oral Surgery at University College Hospital. We continued to take these sailing holidays long after we had left the Eastman and taken up consultancies and professorships elsewhere and only stopped when the Professor's eyesight began to fail and he started attempting to ram lighthouses!

It became very obvious to me that the low standards of teaching in oral surgery in undergraduate dental schools were, in part at least, due to a lack of textbooks on the subject. I decided to try to remedy these deficiencies by writing a trilogy of 'toddler's guides'. From a publisher's point of view there is little money to be made from publishing dental textbooks due to the small size of the potential market. The main specialist publisher in the field was a small family firm in Bristol, John Wright and Sons, and I sought an interview with their Publishing Manager, Mr Owens. He was a kindly man who listened patiently to my ideas for a small book entitled *The Extraction of Teeth* and then equally patiently explained the facts of life in the real world to me. Despite these he agreed to publish the work albeit on a profit sharing agreement under which I would not receive any royalties until all the costs of a run of three thousand copies had been met. I readily agreed for my aim was not to make money but to produce a teaching tool specifically designed to ease the load upon clinical teachers such as myself. To this end I deliberately limited the text to basic principles, avoided references and, believing that a good illustration is worth a thousand words, employed a medical artist to produce a series of line drawings from my rough sketches. I was delighted when the book appeared first in hardback and then as a paperback, for Mr Owens and his colleagues had taken great pains to implement my ideas, the typeface was clearly printed on good quality paper, pictures such as radiographic images were sharply reproduced and illustrations faced the relevant text. The book received favourable reviews and after a few months I received my first royalties and an invitation from Mr Owens to write the other two books that I had mentioned to him.

One day a gentleman called to see me and introduced himself as Oliver Graham Jones, the Veterinary Officer to the London Zoo in which he had established a veterinary hospital. He explained to me that vets specialised according to animal species unlike doctors who specialise according to anatomical and physiological systems. Quite obviously there were few vets specialising in captive wild animals that he could consult about problem cases. Thus he had come to rely on the goodwill and expertise of medical colleagues. He told me that he had a spider monkey named Chico with a severe facial deformity and asked me to come to the Zoo hospital and see him. This I did and having diagnosed the condition as Fibrous Dysplasia on clinical grounds took a surgical specimen for histological examination and some blood for serum electrolyte determination. Ivor Kramer confirmed that the histological appearances were compatible with my clinical diagnosis. Professor Dennis Baron of the Royal Free Hospital Medical School, one of my teachers at the Middlesex, determined the serum electrolyte levels but reported that he could not find any normal levels for spider monkeys in the literature to compare them with. He quickly agreed to assist Oliver in his attempts to compile such

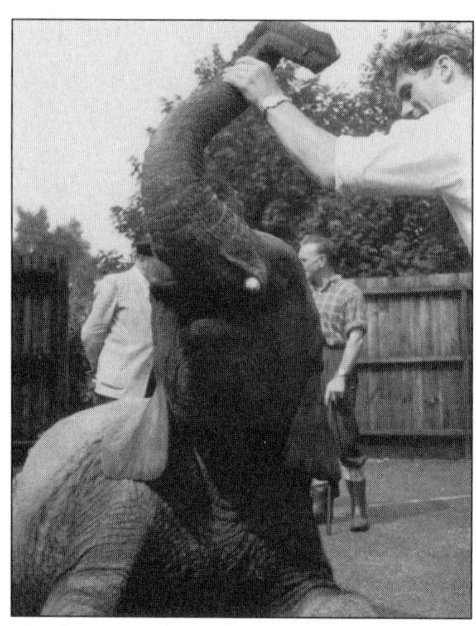

*This elephant's right tusk is unerupted and being embedded in its lip is causing the animal distress.*

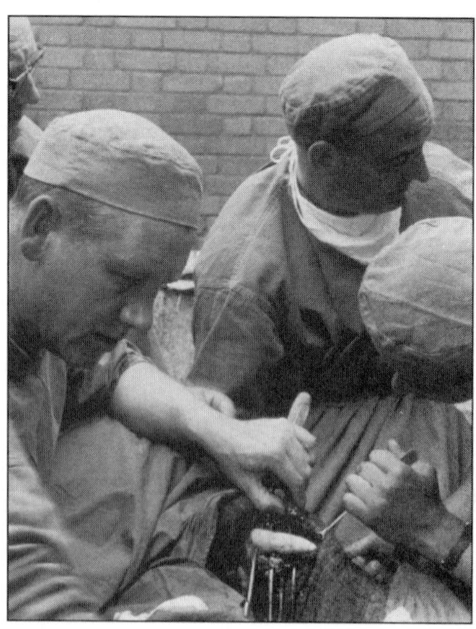

*The tusk has been surgically exposed under local anaesthesia and relaxants in an open air operation. The anaesthetist is Oliver Graham Jones.*

information for all species as a research project. For my part I undertook all the Oral Surgery work in the London Zoo hospital on a voluntary basis for over a decade as a part time hobby and operated on animals large and small on both an outpatient and an inpatient basis until Oliver had to resign due to ill health having caught meningitis in Moscow when attempting to persuade a panda to mate.

About a year after I had returned to the Eastman, Heather and I decided to have a family and I was delighted when she told me that she was pregnant. Little did I know what was in store for us. Heather was in her mid thirties and had almost every known complication of pregnancy including eclampsia, a breech presentation and obstructed labour. I had arranged for her to be confined at the Middlesex and carefully chosen the obstetrician and midwifery sister who would look after her. My confidence in them was misplaced for her labour was badly mishandled. After ten agonising hours I was asked whether I wanted my wife or my baby. I replied that I thought that such questions were only asked in B movies not in my Alma Mater and that I would never forgive them if anything happened to Heather. I never have, despite the fact that both survived a difficult forceps delivery, for Heather's health was wrecked and Timothy John was badly bruised. Heather had always had a tendency to back problems and slipped a disc during labour. She was doubly incontinent for six weeks and breastfed Tim despite being in a plaster jacket. Not surprisingly she went into a severe puerperal depression which lasted for many months. She was to be plagued with both recurrent problems with her spine and repeated bouts of severe depression for the remaining four decades of her life. Needless to say we decided that I would never have the daughter that I had always wanted. Why, oh why, was Timothy John not born by Caesarean section?

In those days senior registrar appointments were made for a limited term and I, in common with my fellow Senior Registrars, was becoming increasingly concerned that no vacancies for consultant posts worthy of the name had been advertised for almost three years. We were poorly paid and had no reserves to fall back on if and when we became unemployed and I now had three mouths to feed in addition to helping to support my widowed mother who had retired when my uncle's practice was sold. A few months after Tim arrived Sir William asked me if I had seen the advertisement for the first Chair in Oral Surgery in the UK which had been established in King's College, Newcastle upon Tyne by the University of Durham. When I told him that I had he enquired why I had not asked him to act as one of my referees. I told him that I had not applied for the post as it was well known that more than twenty established consultants had done so. He told me that he felt I should apply and, if appointed, put my ideas on undergraduate education into practice. By this time Heather, though still convalescent, was almost herself again and when I discussed the matter with her was adamant that I should apply saying that I had only the cost of a postage stamp to lose! I did so and was delighted to be invited for interview for I thought that when one of the established consultants was appointed I had a good chance of getting his job.

I travelled up to Newcastle on the train in atrocious weather. The train halted at the Gateshead end of the railway bridge over the Tyne and I looked down upon a shipbreakers yard. For anyone who loves the sea and ships there can be few more depressing sights. When we arrived at North Road

Station both it and all the buildings around it were black and grimy in the pouring rain. My heart sank for like most southerners this was my picture of the north. I found it so depressing that I went to the enquiries office to find out the time of the next train back to London only to be told that I had just missed one and had more than two hours to wait. So I put my case in the left luggage office, turned up the collar of my trenchcoat and walked around the town. I was pleasantly surprised with what I saw despite the pouring rain. I was impressed with the architecture of Grey Street and the situation of the Royal Victoria Infirmary sitting as it does on the edge of the Town Moor. Knowing that if I did not attend the interview I would not only offend my chiefs but have to pay my train fare, I went back to the station, retrieved my case and checked into the Royal Turk's Head Hotel where after a bath and an excellent fish and chip dinner I had an early night.

The next morning I was shown around both the Sutherland Dental School and the Dental Department of the RVI by Professor (later Sir) Robert Bradlaw. The RVI facility was housed in 'temporary' huts erected during the First World War and the equipment was just as antiquated, all the dental chairs having elaborately carved wooden seats! Professor Bradlaw told me that it had housed the Dental School until the Sutherland Dental School was opened just before the Second World War. He also told me of the ambitious rebuilding plans that the University had approved and hoped soon to implement. The interviews were held in the afternoon and I learned that five other candidates had also been invited to attend. As all my training posts had been obtained in open competition after interview I was familiar with the system and knew that there would always be hostile questioning from those members of the committee who favoured appointing other candidates. Such a person's questions were designed to highlight one's shortcomings and I guessed that, as I was only thirty-four years old, and being fair haired with a pale complexion looked even younger and was only a mere Senior Registrar that I was going to have a lively time!

The Appointments Committee was a large one with the Vice Chancellor, Dr Bosanquet, in the Chair. The Professor of Children's Dentistry was sitting on the extreme right of the committee and was invited to open the questioning. I knew nothing of the University politics in Newcastle and so was totally unaware of his opposition to the Chair being advertised in the first place, and doubly qualified dentists holding the Fellowship rather than a higher University degree in the second. He glowered at me and asked brusquely, 'How old are you?' When I replied that I was in my thirty-fifth year he snapped, 'Well you don't look it!' and sat back, his demolition job done. I was incensed at his lack of courtesy but quietly asked the Vice Chancellor, who was visibly uncomfortable, if I could comment. When he agreed I said that I did not understand the purpose of the question but that if it was designed to illustrate that I was too young for the job I would submit that this was a matter of mental maturity and not of calendar age. Other members of the committee asked me a few routine questions exhibiting the usual courtesies as they did so. As is usual the chairman asked me if I had any questions and when I answered in the negative, told me that the University would let all the candidates know their decision in about one week. I then left wondering where a consultancy would become vacant when its present occupant was appointed to the Chair. In my opinion the favourite for the job was John McCagie, an old friend, who was a Consultant at Stoke Mandeville Hospital and in charge of the teaching of Oral Surgery at the Royal Dental Hospital, for not only was he a surgical Fellow of a Royal College as well as a dental Fellow, but he had worked previously at the Newcastle General Hospital and was married to a lady who was reputed to have family connections in the city. We travelled back to London together and had an excellent dinner, a bottle of wine and a few drinks during the journey. Thus I arrived home having drink taken, itching to tell Heather all my news. Before I could do so she said, 'You've got the job'. I told her we would have news in a week or so. This conversation was repeated a couple of times before she told me that she had answered the telephone and a voice said, 'This is Wobert Bwadlaw, (he had a speech impediment), get your husband to buy you a new hat, you'll need it in Newcastle,' and put the phone down before she could speak. My first reaction was that someone was playing a practical joke on us but I told her all that had happened and added that I had reservations about taking the job even if it was offered to me.

The next morning I was operating with Sir William and was already changed into surgical dress and scrubbing up when he walked into the Scrub Up Room and said, 'Good morning, Professor,' much to the surprise of the others around. Whilst operating he seldom spoke but on this occasion unusually he talked and told me that Professor Bradlaw had telephoned him and told him all about the interview adding that my calm and courteous response to extreme and provocative rudeness had delighted both him and most other members of the committee and had undoubtedly got me the job. When the operating list was over we had lunch together and I told him the full story and detailed the reservations that I had. The most important of these was whether Heather would find happiness in the north east for whilst she had made a good recovery she was far from being her old self again. Alan Mack, who had been a student senior to me at the Royal was the Professor of Prosthetics in Newcastle and lived in a farmhouse near Heddon on the Wall and so it was arranged for Heather to spend a week with Alan and his wife Marjorie and their family during which they agreed to show her around. She was fortunate for weather and she loved the area and returned to London very enthusiastic about the move.

Having sought and obtained various assurances concerning facilities, hospital bed allocations and anaesthetic cover I wrote accepting the Chair and we spent the three months notice that I had to give carefully planning every aspect of the move. In the event it was an absolute disaster. The long drive up the A1 in my little Morris Minor went very well and Tim was very well behaved for the whole journey and we spent the night in the Royal Turks Head Hotel in good spirits. It had been arranged for us to move into a four hundred year old cottage in Spital Tongues, a small village on the Town Moor, and we went to see it the next morning. It had been unoccupied for some time and although it had recently been cleaned up was sorely in need of renovation. This having been promised we sat in the car awaiting the arrival of our furniture for the whole day, finally going back to the hotel as dusk fell to find a message waiting for us to say that the furniture van would arrive the next day. The frustrating wait had been a considerable strain on my convalescent wife who had to look after our small son in cramped circumstances throughout it. Next morning a furniture van that we had never seen before arrived at the cottage at about midday. On questioning we learned that the van into which our home had been loaded had been involved in an accident on the A1 and that all our furniture and personal possessions had had to be transferred into another vehicle during a rainstorm. Worse was to come for as the men carried our three piece suite into the small lounge/living room the floor collapsed revealing a cellar half full of water. We later learned that the floor was riddled with dry rot and that the chains attached to the walls of the cellar had been used to restrain inmates when the property had been part of a bedlam. The bedrooms were habitable, the toilets, though ancient, still flushed and we could use the kitchen if we walked on planks across the remains of the lounge floor, although the elderly gas stove was in such a state that we could only use the rings on the top of it. After an excellent take away fish and chip meal we went to bed absolutely exhausted. Next morning I contacted Professor Bradlaw who quickly organised some emergency repairs for us and so we spent the next few days consorting with workmen. Not surprisingly Heather's health began to deteriorate and caused me great concern for although Tim was very good he needed a great deal of attention.

## Chapter Six

# Life in Newcastle

I WAS DUE TO start work on the 1st April but declined to do so on All Fools Day for obvious reasons, and so reported for duty on the 2nd only to be told by the Bursar that it had been decided that because of my age my starting salary would be four annual increments below the advertised minimum salary of two thousand pounds per annum. As there were already ten increments in the advertised salary scale this meant a very considerable reduction in my career earnings. I told the Bursar that if this was the way the University conducted relations with its staff I did not want to be part of it and walked back to the Dental School to acquaint Professor Bradlaw with my decision to telephone Professor Wilkinson to ask for my old job back. Both of us knew that he had opposed my acceptance of the Chair and offered me a Senior Lectureship at the Eastman. He met me in the Hall and gave me coffee whilst the Vice Chancellor was contacted. A message was then received from the Senior Registrar in Oral Surgery at the Royal Victoria Infirmary saying that three patients with multiple injuries including facial fractures resulting from a road traffic accident had arrived in the Casualty Department and my presence there was requested. I spent the rest of the day participating in their treatment ably assisted by Peter Bradnum, the Senior Registrar, Neil Gough, the Resident House Officer and Harry Charlton, the Maxillofacial Dental Technician, none of whom had I met before. At the end of a long and challenging day we were joined by Professor Bradlaw who asked me not to telephone Professor Wilkinson as he had sorted matters out. As I was anxious to return to Spital Tongues for I knew that Heather would be wondering what had happened to me I readily agreed and arranged to meet him the next morning. When I got home I found Heather in some distress for she had been alone with Tim, except for the workmen all day and had not eaten. However, several cups of tea and a hot snack later she began to relax and I decided not to burden her with the day's woes.

As the days progressed I soon realised the magnitude of the problems to be solved. The Dental School was admitting seventy students in each year of the five year course and although I was not called upon to teach them during their first two years my teaching load was a formidable one. The courses in local anaesthesia, exodontia, oral surgery and oral medicine were completely unplanned, the clinical practices were antediluvian and the standards of patient care unacceptable. All the senior staff in the department were elderly general dental practitioners none of whom had received any formal postgraduate training and all but one of them only attended the hospital on two half days each week. None of them were on call out of hours. The one lecturer post in the department was vacant, there was one registrar who was merely being used as a pair of hands and had had no formal postgraduate education and the housemen were on rotation and spent only six weeks of their six months appointment in the Extraction Room before moving on to another department.

I set about remedying all these deficiencies despite being extremely busy in the Royal Victoria Infirmary. The

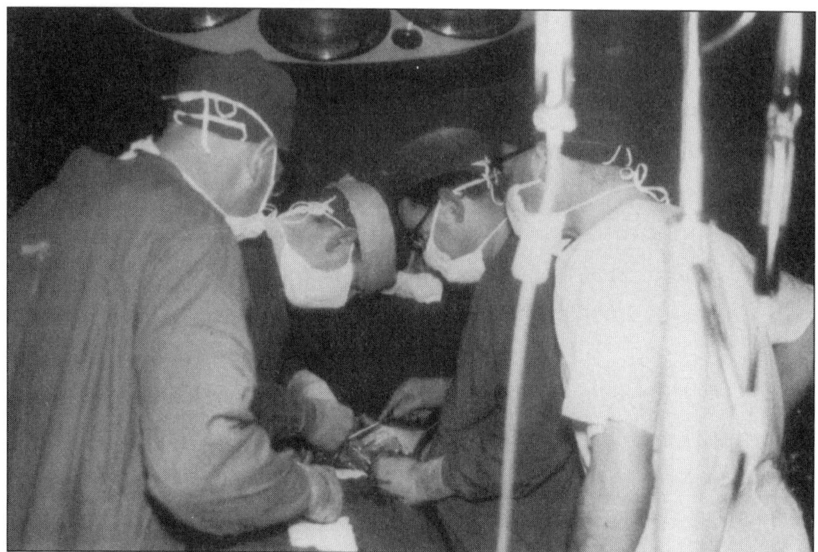

*Operating in the RVI, Newcastle, wearing a sweat band as usual. The first assistant is the late Peter Bradnum, my Senior Registrar at the time.*

Registrar was an excellent fellow, Alex MacGregor, who whilst very conscious that he had only made a partial recovery from a facial palsy was keen to train as an oral surgeon. With the enthusiastic co-operation of the teachers in Oral Anatomy and Oral Physiology I set up an after hours course in the basic medical sciences for my Senior Registrar and Registrar and any other member of junior staff who wished to attend so that they could prepare for the Primary dental fellowship. The vacant lecturer's post was advertised and I was fortunate enough to recruit Lester Kay, a doubly qualified registrar with the dental Fellowship with whom I had worked at the Eastman and so knew to be ideally suited to be an undergraduate teacher. In the following years he was a tower of strength and was not only idolised and greatly loved by the students, but was the mainstay of the research activities in the Department obtaining the degree of Master of Dental Surgery for an outstanding thesis on Pericoronitis. I was his supervisor for this project and was absolutely delighted though not surprised when he was awarded this accolade which, being the equivalent of a Mastership in Surgery, was ranked higher than a Doctor of Philosophy degree in the University of Durham. Both Peter Bradnum and Alex MacGregor passed the Primary Fellowship at their first attempt and so Lester and I organised an out of hours course for the Final Fellowship examination for them on which they were joined by a jovial Dubliner named Frank Allen, who had replaced Neil Gough as Resident Dental Officer. All three passed the Final Examination at the first attempt thus confirming my views about both their ability and potential and became full members of my young and enthusiastic team.

I was working for very long hours and so was unable to spend as much time with Heather and Tim as I would have wished. I shall always be grateful to Shirley Bradnum, Peter's new wife, who was a nursing sister at the RVI, for seeing my concerns she took them both under her wing. Unfortunately despite all her efforts Heather became deeply depressed once again. Her mother, a widow for a number of years had remarried and lived in the village of Landrake, near Saltash in Cornwall, immediately offered to look after Tim until Heather could do so and so I decided to take him down to her. Shirley prepared food and drink for him, he had been weaned by this time, and Heather moved into the Bradnum home. I drove Tim across country, feeding him, potting him and moving him occasionally from his carrycot on the backseat into a baby seat as we went along. The journey took sixteen hours and I was absolutely exhausted when my beloved mother in law, Winifred Mary, greeted us on our arrival and took over, for I slept for sixteen hours that night. She looked after him splendidly until Heather and I were able to collect him about six months later, indeed by that time he seemed to regard us as strangers for the first few hours.

During the intervening period I had been looking for a new home and after several months had at last found a very nice family house which had just been built in Tynemouth in Northumberland. The trouble was that it was priced at £5,500 and I had been brought up to believe that one's mortgage should never be more than twice one's annual income and so I dithered until Heather was well enough to take an interest in solving our housing problems. Mr Moffat of the Medical Insurance Agency had offered to provide a 100% mortgage against endowment insurance and assured me that although finances would be tight for a while I could afford to buy the house. As soon as she was well enough I took Heather to see the house which she loved at first sight and she urged me to take the plunge. To this end she teamed up with Mr Moffat and a bottle of sherry to persuade me to sign the necessary papers and so make one of the best decisions of my life. We could not afford to furnish all the rooms or buy carpets for several months but we moved the furniture that we had into the lounge, kitchen and two bedrooms leaving the other rooms empty. We then collected Timothy John from Cornwall and started to live as a family once more.

Heather was an excellent cook and homemaker and soon made us cosy although I had to employ Elsie, a buxom young miner's wife, to do the heavier work. She was a typical warm hearted and generous north easterner who adored Tim and soon became one of the family, leaving us only when she started a family of her own. Heather also always had green fingers and found great pleasure in creating a garden from scratch which was soon the envy of all our neighbours.

Professionally I was working long hours and being a single handed consultant was on call continuously, often being called out to treat patients with maxillofacial injuries on two or three nights in one week. My young colleagues in the department, including the maxillofacial dental technician, Harry Charlton, soon became an enthusiastic, able and industrious team and working together we transformed the standards of patient care despite the inadequacies in both equipment and facilities of the department which as previously mentioned was housed in a 'temporary hut' erected on the RVI site during the First World War. The RVI was an extremely busy hospital with an outstanding consultant staff in almost every speciality who were most co-operative and supportive and combined clinics were soon established with the plastic surgeons, oncologists and dermatologists who were interested in lesions of the oral mucosa. The paediatric department under Professor Donald Court was a centre of excellence and housed the Regional Centre for haemophilia. I was appalled at the incidence of untreated dental disease in such patients which often precipitated so-called 'dental crises' as tooth extraction became unavoidable and was complicated by torrential haemorrhage which was extremely difficult to control and arrest often requiring blood transfusion, and so I attempted to set up a system of regular dental inspections and care with the emphasis on the prevention of dental disease. Unfortunately quite a few patients and their parents failed to appreciate the value of such a service and so uptake was slow.

It was also difficult to find paedodontists capable of undertaking this work load and prepared to do so.

Although I was extremely happy working in such an environment I was often aware of my own inadequacies and especially so when exhausted. On one occasion I was called out in the middle of the night to treat a coalminer who had sustained a severe maxillofacial injury in a mine accident. This was the major injury amongst several others and so I was called upon to decide whether to operate immediately or to resuscitate him first. Intensive care and resuscitation units had not been established at that time. I decided to operate and the patient died in the Anaesthetic Room before being wheeled into the Operating Theatre. I arrived home early in the morning too late to go to bed, had a bath and went to work as usual. That night I was called out again to find another miner with almost identical injuries. In view of my experience the previous night I decided to resuscitate him first and he died in the early hours of the morning. I slept for an hour or two in my office and first thing next morning telephoned Sir William to say that I did not feel up to the job. He asked me some technical details and then told me to stop thinking I was Jesus Christ for no one could have done any better. He advised me to get some sleep and to then attend the post-mortem examinations. This I did and the findings of the Pathologist confirmed his views.

Whilst I loved working in the RVI I did not enjoy working in the Dental Hospital where my efforts to raise the standards of patient care and undergraduate education in my discipline were constantly obstructed. About six months after I arrived in Newcastle the Dean, Professor Robert Bradlaw, had left to become Dean of the Postgraduate Dental School in the Eastman Dental Hospital in London, and in the next few months the atmosphere in the Dental Hospital was clouded by a competition between the Professors of Conservative Dentistry and of Children's Dentistry for the Deanship. Both had supporters and opponents and political manoeuvring and lobbying were intense. My refusal to become involved in this and support either of them against the other was deeply resented by both. They then came to believe, quite erroneously, that my actions indicated a desire to become Dean myself. Nothing could have been further from the truth as I was already desperately over committed, a fact that must have been obvious to even the most casual observer. Nevertheless they went to great pains to make my life as difficult as possible and to sour my relationships with my colleagues with moderate success. The appointment of a successor to Professor Bradlaw was extremely badly handled by the University and the unpleasantness went on for months during which morale in the Dental Hospital and School rapidly deteriorated. The matter was finally decided by making one the Dean and the other the Director of the Dental Hospital thus perpetuating the divisions in both institutions.

Despite all these problems the Department of Oral Surgery prospered and standards of patient care and undergraduate teaching were transformed. Much of the credit for these improvements belongs to Lester Kay for his superhuman efforts which overcame all the obstacles placed in our path. His reward was to be denied promotion two years in succession by the Dean despite being better qualified, more experienced and senior to others who were promoted. Unfortunately for my department, Professor Bradlaw heard of this and immediately offered Lester the post of Senior Lecturer and Honorary Consultant at the Eastman and so we lost the services of a delightful colleague and the best teacher of Oral Surgery to undergraduates that I have ever known.

I worked in Newcastle for eight years the first four of which were in King's College of the University of Durham, and the last four in the University of Newcastle upon Tyne which King's College became. I had the doubtful distinction of being the only Professor in Newcastle to vote against the division of the University of Durham and later to oppose the changes in university education proposed in the Robbin's report. I have no regrets about this as I remain convinced that both events led to the decline in university standards which has since occurred. The atmosphere in the Dental School and Hospital continued to deteriorate and some very able younger members of staff looked for pastures new. Newcastle's loss was the profession's gain, for colleagues such as Peter Burke, John Farrell, Alan Mack and Freddie Hopper had distinguished careers elsewhere. Both the Dean and the Director continued to make difficulties for me and, in the Committees of the School, Faculty and University constantly referred to me as 'the boy Professor'.

Fortunately as head of the Dental Department of the RVI I had a seat on the Medical Advisory Committee of the United Newcastle upon Tyne Hospitals. This important and influential body was chaired by Professor Edgar Pask, the Professor of Anaesthesia, and was attended by many colleagues with national and international reputations in their disciplines. 'Gar' Pask was a remarkable man and more of a physiological researcher than a clinician. He was convinced that the then standard Board of Trade life jacket drowned unconscious persons by allowing their faces to go under the surface of the water. Having been frustrated by officialdom he decided to prove his point in the most dramatic way. He arranged to be taken out in a lifeboat and dumped into the sea, after being given a muscle relaxant drug to paralyse him, wearing a BOT lifejacket. The whole exercise was filmed and clearly demonstrated that his opinions were correct. He risked his life to prove his point. Little wonder then that when the Seahouses lifeboat was lost its replacement was called the *Edgar Pask*.

Such was the calibre of the chairman, who, as I took my seat in one particular MAC meeting, signalled to me to look at the paper 'laid on the table' in front of me. This I did and to my surprise found that it was a letter signed by both the Dean and the Director expressing the view that the dental representation on the MAC was over generous and should be reduced from three seats to two. I signalled to the chairman that I knew nothing about this proposal. Under Any Other Business he invited the signatories to the letter to speak one after the other and this they did at some length. He then pointed out to the MAC that I had not signed the letter and asked if I had any comments to make. I said that not having had time to think about the matter there was little that I could say about it but that there might be some merit in it. However if there was I, as the sole representative of the RVI dental department on the MAC, would be happy to let the Dean and Director decide which of them should resign. A titter went around the table and the proposal was hurriedly withdrawn.

This was a turning point in my career in Newcastle for during the next few days a number of senior colleagues from the RVI and Medical School including Gar Pask came to see me and to tell me that I could rely on their backing and support as they now realised the difficulties that I was working under. They were as good as their word and during the next two or three years the RVI dental department was refurbished. I was allowed to use their beds to admit and treat emergency admissions and Newcastle came to be regarded as developing into a centre of excellence in Oral Surgery. The junior staff prospered and having obtained their Fellowships at the first attempt began to publish articles in learned journals and to read papers at scientific congresses. Money was found to establish a full time consultant post and we were joined by Tony Parnell, an old friend of mine from Royal days. He laboured long and hard in both the Dental Hospital and the old Freeman's Fields Hospital for several years before accepting an invitation to fill the Chair of Oral Surgery in the University of London, Ontario, Canada.

We were always busy and time passed quickly. I published 'Minor Oral Surgery' and was awarded the Cartwright Prize of the Royal College of Surgeons of England for an essay in which I detailed my clinical research into surgical aids to prosthetics. This prize, which can only be awarded to medically qualified dentists once every five years, had not been awarded since the 1920s when my mentor, Sir William, had been the last recipient. He was ecstatic when I won the prize and a few months later was awarded the Master of Dental Surgery degree in the University of Durham. I was much in demand as a lecturer and was elected to the Board of the Faculty of Dentistry of the RCS of England, as a Founder Fellow of both the British and the International Associations of Oral Surgeons and became one of the first examiners and recipients of the Fellowship of the Faculty of Dentistry of the RCS in Ireland. I was also elected as

President of the Oral Surgery Club of Great Britain and was privileged to host a meeting in Newcastle during which we had four operating theatres running at once in which all members of the unit displayed their skills. I chaired an overseas meeting seeing what our French Colleagues in Lyon were doing. I published about twenty papers in learned journals as well as the textbooks. In addition to examining in both Newcastle and Dublin I served as External Examiner in the University of Baghdad, Iraq, and read papers at Conferences in Rome, Paris, Dublin, London, Limerick, Copenhagen and Bergen.

Some of these trips were not without incident, for example my trip to Copenhagen. Most British participants in the 2nd International Conference on Oral Surgery travelled by air but living in Newcastle I caught the ferry to Esbjerg and then the train to Copenhagen arriving an hour or two after them. When I got to my hotel I found absolute chaos in the foyer for due to computer errors most rooms, including mine, had been triple booked. The Hall Porter told me that I could probably find a bed at a hotel of similar standard situated close by if I acted quickly. I did and was relieved to find its foyer empty except for the receptionist whom I asked if he had a vacant room. He nodded his head and asked how long I planned to stay and appeared surprised when I said one week. I asked the price and he replied that it depended upon the services that I required. I replied just bed and breakfast and he then quoted me a very reasonable price, which after inspecting the room and finding it to be en suite and spotlessly clean I accepted. After having a bath and changing my clothes I went to the opening ceremony of the Conference in the City Hall, a most impressive occasion in which the excellent food and drink were eaten to the accompaniment of long Viking horns. Feeling tired after my long journey I decided to have an early night. On returning to the hotel I was surprised to find a rugby scrum in progress in the foyer but fought my way through it, got my key and went to bed, and was soon sound asleep. In the early hours of the morning I woke up to find an inebriated Frenchman minus his trousers in my room. With some difficulty I persuaded him that he was in the wrong room and he left apologising profusely. I locked the door and went back to sleep until woken by my travelling alarm clock at 7.00 a.m. I was surprised to find that I was the only guest taking breakfast in a large dining room. I was served an excellent breakfast by a rather haggard and blowsy peroxide blonde, cleaned my teeth and went to the Congress Centre to register. The charming young lady receptionist enquired whether I was one of the many unfortunates whose accommodation arrangements had gone awry. I said that whilst I was, there was no problem as I had managed to get a room in a hotel in a nearby street and showed her the hotel card. On reading it she went bright scarlet and rushed into the room behind her. She returned accompanied by the President of both the International Association and the Congress, Sir Terence Ward of East Grinstead fame, an old friend and colleague of mine. He was grinning from ear to ear as he told me that I had booked into the most famous brothel in Copenhagen if not the whole of Scandinavia. The receptionist then offered me alternative accommodation some distance from the Conference Centre which I declined. The Scientific Programme commenced in the afternoon with a Symposium on Pre Prosthetic Surgery in which I was one of the keynote speakers. The Chairman was Sir Terence who conducted affairs in his own inimitable manner. When it came to my turn to speak he introduced me as the youngest clinical professor in Great Britain, which I believe I was for my first six years in Newcastle, and then added that in order to flaunt this fact I had booked into the Hotel X, that notorious house of ill repute, for the entire week of the conference. The international audience of more than a thousand colleagues went into gales of laughter, which due to the simultaneous translation came in waves and was therefore prolonged. I was laughing as much as anyone as I mounted the rostrum and delivered my paper. Later in the conference I delivered a second paper after Sir Terence had said that I appeared to be standing up well and congratulated me on my stamina. I did not change hotels for whilst I had my suspicions I was treated with both courtesy and respect throughout my stay and left having saved money on my accommodation.

I managed to contract viral meningitis after performing emergency surgery on a patient with the disease, despite working under full aseptic conditions, about halfway through my sojourn in Newcastle. I am atopic and have an allergy to penicillin amongst many others. Unfortunately the doctor who treated me whilst I was unconscious ignored the warning on my case notes and gave me penicillin. It was not indicated, nor of the slightest value in treatment but worsened my condition and delayed my recovery by some weeks, during which my bed was filled with scales of skin. Nevertheless I made a complete recovery and remained in the highest Army medical category 'Forward everywhere'.

Towards the end of my time in Newcastle I was going to London at least once a week for meetings at the Royal College of Surgeons and the British Dental Association for I had been elected as the sole representative of the English

Provincial Dental Hospitals on the newly formed autonomous Hospital and Specialists Committee about which more anon. I also continued to operate on demand in the Veterinary Hospital of the London Zoo in Regent's Park and to attend TA training with my own unit whenever I could.

It was my custom to catch a train to Kings Cross at North Road Station at about 6.00 p.m. and to take dinner on the train arriving in London at about 10.00 p.m. I still recall the excellence of the steak and kidney pie on the East Coast Line. I then spent the night in one of the small hotels in or around Russell Square and went to work the next day after an early breakfast usually returning to Newcastle in the evening. I carried on this rather hectic lifestyle for some time but then began to experience acute symptoms during some of the train journeys which led me to believe that I had developed a hiatus hernia. These suspicions were confirmed by the Dean of Medicine, Professor Andrew Lowdon after an extensive radiographic examination had shown that I had what he called the father and mother of a paraoesophageal hiatus hernia. He suggested immediate admission and surgery but fully understood when I told him that I felt bound to honour a commitment to examine in Baghdad the following week as the unfortunate students there had had their course extended by two months to suit my convenience. I flew to Baghdad only to find the temperature 100°F and a sandstorm in progress. I marked the examination papers sitting in a bath of cold water being sprayed with a fine dust via the air conditioning. As requested by my Iraqi colleagues I marked everything at British standard and was greatly impressed by both the calibre of the students and the standards that they achieved under great difficulties and with limited resources. This was largely due to the excellent teaching provided by three young Iraqi colleagues who had done their postgraduate training in the UK where they had obtained both dental fellowships and English wives.

During my last two days in Iraq there was a civil uprising during which a man was lynched in the street alongside the hotel and I was relieved to board the BOAC flight home. I was the only first class passenger and having been recognised by the air hostess, who had been a Dental Surgery Assistant at Guy's when I was an LDS examiner there, was looked after superbly. I arrived home in excellent spirits to find orders to join my TA unit training in a battle training zone in Germany. This I did and managed to complete assault courses and other strenuous training without my hiatus hernia causing me too much trouble. Whilst in Baghdad I had walked along the Ceremonial Way of the Hanging Gardens of Babylon and through the Gateway which I was told was a replica of the original which had been taken to Berlin by German Archaeologists in 1904. A few weeks later during my TA training I spent a weekend in Berlin and went to a museum in East Berlin where I saw not only the original gate but also the head of Nefertiti.

Feeling well on my return to the north east I decided to postpone surgery until we returned from holiday about one month later and so off we went to Sarnen, which borders the lake of that name just above Lake Lucerne in Switzerland. After about one week there I suddenly experienced severe pain in the abdomen and the left side of my chest accompanied by difficulty in swallowing and we decided to fly home immediately. This we did and I was admitted to the RVI as an emergency as soon as I arrived.

Tests showed that my stomach and spleen had passed through the defect in my diaphragm and into my chest and that my left lung had collapsed. Andrew Lowdon had unfortunately had a coronary thrombosis and died a week or two earlier and so I was looked after by his Reader, Frank Walker, who undoubtedly saved my life. During a prolonged operation he removed my spleen which was too swollen to be returned to my abdomen with my stomach, repaired the defect in my diaphragm, drained my chest, performed a vagotomy and a gastrostomy through which I could be fed. I woke up in intensive care doubly incontinent and with transfusions running into all four limbs and cursing myself for my stupidity.

I had been a member of the Committee charged with the task of setting up the Intensive Care Unit in the RVI for the preceding three years. I was the third patient admitted into it and learned more about Intensive Care in the next three days than I had in the preceding three years! I found that I was unable to stop myself slipping down the bed which I constantly dirtied and so asked for a 'donkey', that is a bolster in a sheet placed across the bottom of the bed, on which I could place my feet and control my body position. My old friend, the amiable Sister Murphy who was in charge of the unit, laughingly told me that donkey's were prehistoric and had not been used for years. Nevertheless I persisted with my request and so she summoned the assistance of Matron who told me how old fashioned a Professor I was and that all that I had to do was to press the button on the hand control beside me and the nurses would be delighted to heave me up the bed. I looked at each of the drips in my four limbs in turn and quietly asked her whether she expected me to press the button with my 'one per cent' (penis) and so I got my donkey.

The hospital staff of every grade could not have been kinder to me, the porters shaved me daily, the electricians rigged up both TV and radio for me and as soon as I could swallow again the Catering Staff offered to cook me anything I fancied at any hour of the day or night. I had taught all the nurses during their preliminary training school (PTS) days and they could not do enough for me. My special nurse was Nurse Bookless who gave me devoted care although being a deeply religious person herself was very disturbed when I refused pastoral visits from priests of all denominations. After several weeks the time came for me to be discharged but unfortunately Heather was not well enough for me to go home. Stella, the newly wed wife of my Plastic Surgery colleague, Ian Wilson, took me into their home and cared for me excellently which surprised everyone, for she was a glamour girl, an actress and television presenter who had her own show on Tyne Tees Television. Heather recovered sufficiently after a week or two for me to return to Tynemouth where I gradually regained my strength and energy. My secretary, Vera Dyer, helped me to learn to walk again when she took me out and about and after about six weeks I was able to walk unaided. Fortunately I had an experienced and competent Senior Registrar, Russell Hopkins and an excellent Senior House Officer, Peter McAndrew, at the time who 'looked after the shop' very competently in my absence. I returned to work part time about two months after surgery but was not fit enough to operate for another four months.

When I accepted the Chair I did so on the promise of twelve beds in the RVI for Oral Surgery, but on taking up the appointment found that I only had four borrowed beds in the ENT ward for my exclusive use and that no request for the promised beds had been included in the Quinquennial Estimates which had been prepared before my arrival. The heavy emergency workload of the Department meant that at any one time I could have as many as twenty patients housed in other consultants' beds all over the hospital. My colleagues naturally expected us to inconvenience them as little as possible and to fit into their operating schedules wherever it was practicable to do so – a nightmare organisational headache. Therefore I was both relieved and delighted when it was agreed that remedying this deficiency was to have top priority in the new Dental Quinquennial Estimates. Unfortunately these were finalised whilst I was in Intensive Care and so I did not discover that the request for the promised beds had been deleted from the estimates by my senior dental colleagues during my absence and without consultation. I was incensed and sought interviews with both the Vice Chancellor and the Dean of Medicine only to learn that the estimates had already been submitted.

Whilst I was in hospital I had received a letter from Ben Fickling, one of the Consultants I had served as a Senior House Officer at the Royal. I was surprised to hear from him as I had found him extremely fussy and difficult to work with and we were never close. In essence the letter reminded me that he was now the Senior Surgeon at the Royal and had been adamantly opposed to the creation of a Chair of Oral Surgery there. However the School Council and the Medical Committee of the Hospital had agreed that such a Chair should be established and he accepted that decision and felt that, as Senior Surgeon, it was his duty to ensure that someone of calibre should be appointed to it. Thus, in conversation with John Hovell, he was saddened to learn that he had tried to interest me in the appointment repeatedly and I had said that I was not interested in it. On reflection he had remembered that we had not enjoyed working together and he wondered if this fact had influenced my decision. He asked me to apply when the post was advertised and pledged his 100% support and co-operation if I were appointed. The letter of a very big man as future events were to prove. As soon as I was able I replied telling him about my condition and promising to consider the matter when I was fit.

The Chair was advertised about two weeks after I had learned that I was condemned to continue coping with the chaotic bed situation for at least another five years, and so Heather and I discussed the matter for days on end. I was very happy working in the RVI and pleased with the substantial progress that I and the excellent team that I had recruited and trained had made in the eight years that I had been in Newcastle. On the other hand I found it difficult to work with colleagues that I neither respected nor trusted. Heather and I had a nice comfortable home and a good family life, we enjoyed living in the north east and Tim was happy in Newlands, his prep school and both he and Heather had a wide circle of friends. I did not relish the idea of throwing away the results of eight years hard work and starting all over again nor leaving my young colleagues and my students. On the other hand I was having to make the long journeys to and from London more and more frequently as my various commitments there constantly increased. After much heart searching we decided that I should apply. This I did and after interview was offered the

Chair and given one month to make my mind up. I returned to Newcastle and sought meetings with the Vice Chancellor and the Registrar of the University in which I explained the situation and asked that something be done to ease the chaotic bed situation. Weeks passed and nothing happened and so I wrote to the University of London accepting the Chair and submitted my resignation to the University of Newcastle. Only then was there a response during which I was exhorted to stay but I decided that it was too little too late and time to move on and so I did.

## Chapter Seven

# Back at my Alma Mater

My first problem was to find somewhere to live for I was to be allocated beds in St George's Hospitals at both Hyde Park Corner and Tooting and St Thomas's Hospital and the Lambeth Hospital and was required to live within seven miles of all of them. As the various hospitals were widely separated this limited my choice of location severely. I had never lived south of the Thames and so did not know where to look for property. When I finally found a suitable town house being built in South Croydon I was astounded at the price and had to arrange for an additional mortgage. As correctly foreseen by both Heather and Mr Moffat I was able to sell the house in Tynemouth quite easily and for a good price but the new house was about twice as dear. We moved into it only to find defects and deficiencies which made it necessary for us to move out again for one month whilst they were remedied. In some ways it was fortunate that the new Danish furniture that we had ordered did not arrive for three months!

My main base was the Royal Dental Hospital in Leicester Square and I used to commute there on a 'crab and winkle' line via Charing Cross Station from Coombe Road Station which was only two or three hundred yards from my home. This was fortunate for on most days I left home at 7.00 a.m. and returned at about 7.00 p.m. If I worked late I had to return via East Croydon Station which was a twenty minute walk from my home. Thus I saw little of Tim and Heather except at weekends. One thing that Heather and I did not like in the north east was the accent and we went to great lengths to try to prevent Tim from acquiring it and thought that we had succeeded in doing so. Imagine our surprise when I asked him how he liked his new prep school in Purley and he replied, 'Very much, they've even given me a nickname, they all call me Geordie!'

On the work front there was much to do on each of the five sites on which I worked. I had to travel between them on either public transport or on foot as it was not worth taking the car into town. Slowly I built up a good team, raised clinical and teaching standards and initiated clinical research projects. My efforts were hampered by constant reorganisation of the NHS which was accompanied by closures and relocation of both beds and units. Most of the nursing staff in my units were part timers and tied by family commitments to work in particular locations and so there was constant and persistent wastage of nurses familiar with the special demands of the speciality and a constant need to train their successors. I was extremely fortunate to have Ken Ray as a full time Senior Lecturer/Honorary Consultant and, when he left to take up a consultant post in Reading, to have John Towers succeed him. I also had a succession of very able Senior Registrars, including Myer Leonard and Derek Wilson, all of whom went on to become either NHS consultants or Professors. I wrote 'Local Anaesthesia in Dentistry' in co-operation with F. Ivor Whitehead who was in charge of the Oral Surgery department of the new Birmingham Dental Hospital whilst I was an External Examiner there, and published about twenty-five more papers in learned journals whilst working in London. I also acted as an External Examiner in Singapore, Belfast, Dublin, Malta, Melbourne and the Royal Colleges in both London and Dublin as well as being an Internal Examiner in the University of London. I travelled widely lecturing and demonstrating in both Europe and North and South America. Life was very full for I was also becoming more and more involved in the politics of the profession as the British Dental Association fought to keep dental care free at moment of use within the NHS, and I was also rising towards command in the Territorial Army as well as being a member of a plethora of committees. But more of this later.

One of the other problems at the Royal was that there were two factions amongst the staff there, one supporting a unified Department of Restorative Dentistry and the other vehemently opposing it. After prolonged debate in the Dental School Council, long before my arrival at the Royal, the department had been set up replacing the separate departments of Conservative Dentistry and Prosthetics. Unfortunately those opposed to the experiment moved heaven and earth to ensure that it did not succeed and so antagonised many of their colleagues, including the Dean, Professor Raleigh Lucas, the distinguished Oral Pathologist, who devoted most of his time to trying to get people to work together for the good of the institution and the students. He had been an outstanding Dean for twelve years when some five years after my return to the Royal he gave notice of his intention to stand down. It was the custom in the Royal to elect a Vice Dean who took over the Deanship one year later. A very unpleasant polarisation developed between the factions who each had a candidate and being known to be a neutral, I was urged to run for the office. However at the time I was already commanding a major TAVR Unit and leading the profession as Chairman of Council of the British Dental Association and so did not wish to do so. The situation deteriorated and I reluctantly agreed to allow my name to go forward on condition that I would neither electioneer nor lobby and did not want others to do so on my behalf. Not surprisingly, I was not elected in the election which ensued but my relief was short-lived for it emerged that irregularities had occurred and so a second ballot was held in which I was the clear winner and thus condemned to take over the burdens which Raleigh Lucas had carried for so long.

As part of the redevelopment plans of the University the Royal had been linked with both St George's Hospital Medical School and Chelsea College and was to be housed in new buildings on a site in Tooting. Over the preceding two decades there had been many delays and many changes but some progress had been made. At the time that I became Dean the Pre-clinical Departments of the Royal were housed in a magnificent new building in Tooting whilst the Clinical Departments were still housed in a seventy year old building in Leicester Square. Not only did this cause operational difficulties as the two sites were seven miles apart but it also put a considerable strain on the Royal. To make matters worse it was patently obvious that St George's did not have either the resources or teachers to provide an adequate course in Medicine and Surgery for Dental students. They were experiencing great difficulties in rebuilding and appointed a very experienced and capable medical politician, Dr Robert Lowe, as their Dean to get the job done.

At about the same time Sir Keith Joseph, the Secretary of State for Health in the Thatcher Government, introduced a

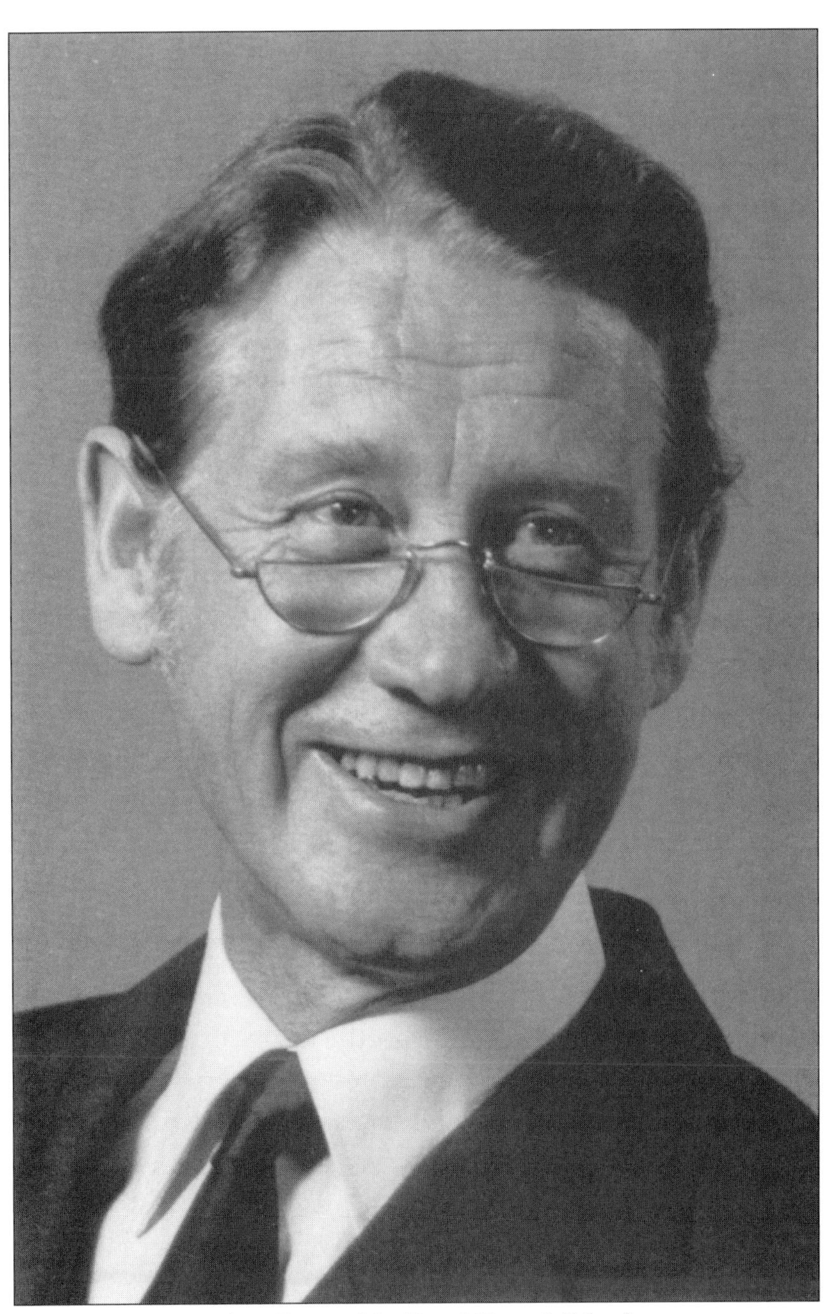

*When Dean of the Royal Dental School.*

disastrous 'reform' of the National Health Service in the mistaken belief that so called 'good management' was an effective substitute for adequate and realistic funding thus complicating a confused situation further. In order to cope with this situation I persuaded the Dental School Council to appoint a Vice Dean to assist me and was fortunate enough to have Harry Blackwood, the Professor of Oral Anatomy, appointed. He was based at Tooting and assumed responsibility for the day to day running of affairs there. I held discussions with the Consultant Staff of St Helier Hospital, a large non teaching hospital in Carshalton, Surrey, which resulted in several of them being appointed as part time Lecturers in the Dental School and their creating an outstanding course in Medicine and Surgery for Dental students. Throughout my Deanship I had excellent relationships with Chelsea College but found Dr Lowe very difficult to deal with. He was ruthless in his efforts to get St George's Hospital and Medical School rebuilt and quite prepared to succeed at the expense of both the Royal and Chelsea College if it became necessary to do so. He was very familiar with the levers of power and used them very effectively to achieve his aims. I had to be constantly on the lookout for developments which might affect the Royal adversely. He was well aware of the divisions which plagued the Royal at that time as well as the many other problems that we were facing and so I devoted much time and energy to acting as a peace maker and trying to get everyone to use the democratic processes to make policy decisions which could be accepted and implemented by all. I was fortunate that the Trust set up at the turn of the century by the colleagues who built the Leicester Square building provided monies for research equipment and used this to help change the climate in the School and get everyone going forward as a team. We also acquired a large house close to Clapham North Underground Station which we converted into living accommodation for students. As Clapham North was on the Northern Line, as were both Tooting and Leicester Square, this did much to ease another long standing problem. Somehow we kept going and were delighted to get excellent reports following quinquennial visitations by inspectors from both the University Grants Committee and the General Dental Council.

About halfway through my tenure of the Deanship of the Royal Heather and a friend were sitting in my boxy old Morris Oxford which was stationary in the middle of the road waiting to turn right when a British Road Services lorry travelling far too fast smashed into the car pushing it a hundred yards down the road. The car was a total write off and Heather's friend in the passenger seat, although wearing a seat belt, collided with the windscreen and some weeks later had a coronary thrombosis and died. Heather sustained multiple injuries breaking both her neck and her back amongst other things. When she regained consciousness in Intensive Care her first words to me were to apologise for being in my car rather than hers. I told her I was delighted that she was for I doubted that we would have been talking if she had been in her little Triumph Herald.

After a stormy few days during which it looked as if I might lose her, her condition suddenly improved and she began to recover. It was a long road which she trod with great fortitude until about six months later she learned to walk again, showing great determination as she did so. Her recovery was never complete and during the next twenty-three years she had many operations including two major operations to remove bony excesses occluding her spinal canal and pressing upon her lumbar nerves causing her agonising pain. The second of these left her with impaired sensation below the waist and difficulty in controlling her natural functions. She was very determined to live as normal a life as was possible and hated anyone to know that she had any disabilities whatsoever. She achieved both objectives much to my surprise although I was amazed at her fortitude and was full of admiration for her courage when she was occasionally over ambitious. She adamantly insisted that I did not give up any of my many offices on her account and, with great determination, was at my side whenever it was expected of her to be there.

In addition to my TA and dental political activities, of which more anon, I acted as University of London Assessor for all the equipment proposals for the dental component of the new Guy's Hospital and School, was a member of the Council and the Board of the Faculty of Dental Surgery of the Royal College of Surgeons of England, the Dental Committee in Dental Surgery of the Joint Committee for Higher Training in Dentistry, the Councils of both the International and British Associations of Oral Surgeons of both of which I was a Founder Fellow and a Trustee of the Royal Army Dental Corps Museum from its foundation.

In June 1976 I was appointed as Chairman of the Dental Academic Advisory Committee of the University of Hong Kong in which capacity I was responsible for the production of the accommodation and equipment schedules and a curriculum for what became the Prince Philip Dental Hospital and School. The University and Polytechnics Grants Committee of Hong Kong wished to introduce dental education at an international standard in Hong Kong in 1979 which, as we were starting absolutely from scratch, was a very tall order, said by many in the field to be completely unrealistic. I disagreed, relished the challenge to do something creative and actually enjoyed commuting between London and Hong Kong for the next two years. The Committee was a small one composed of experts in all relevant fields who came from both England and Hong Kong and were enthusiastic about and wholly committed to the Project. It was a joy to work with them and to marvel at the rapid progress that we made.

This was at a time when both the politicians of all parties and the Trade Unions were reaping havoc in the NHS and the health professionals were having to work harder and harder, and longer and longer to maintain standards and not always succeeding in doing so. I did not enjoy this situation for I felt that the NHS was the greatest social experiment of our time and had been succeeding and slowly but surely, achieving objective after objective until party politics intervened. I still believe this to be true despite the fact that both the NHS and its staff have been a party political football for the past quarter of a century. I was honoured to be elected Centenary President Elect of the British Dental Association to serve with Prince Philip as President of Honour. However it made me think seriously about my future for I was still a young in heart fifty-four year old who loved clinical work, teaching, research and the joy of seeing one's juniors and students succeeding. I have always relished challenge and I felt that I was gradually but inexorably being edged into becoming a pillar of the establishment.

The work of the DAAC was going well and after a year's work we recommended to the University of Hong Kong that it was time to appoint a full time Dean. The University agreed and I spearheaded the search for the right individual but found it impossible to find an experienced Chinese academic capable of doing the job and prepared to accept the challenge. As the months went by the Vice Chancellor, Dr Rayson Huang, began to pressure me to take the job myself and despite realising what I would have to give up in the UK I began to wonder whether this was the chance to do something positive with my life. Over weeks and indeed months Heather and I talked of little else. She was very supportive as always and although looking forward to being the Centenary President's Lady had become increasingly interested in the Hong Kong Dental Project and indeed had accompanied me on one or two of my visits to Hong Kong and met and liked many of the folk there. At that time her medical condition was stable, she was virtually pain free and coping with her disabilities extremely well.

When the invitations to dental supply companies to tender for the equipment for the Dental Hospital and School were issued the Vice Chancellor saw me in London and told me that it was time to make a decision one way or the other if the project was not to be delayed and offered me generous terms and 100% support if I would accept the position. After dithering for a week or two I decided to do so and resign all my offices in the UK. I wrote to him accepting the post on condition that he would allow me a few months in which to put my affairs in the UK in order before I assumed office. This he did by return of post and the deed was done. When the news broke it caused a flutter in the profession and many of my friends and colleagues told me that I had taken leave of my senses. Sir Robert Bradlaw, at that time Dean of the Eastman and President of the General Dental Council, was particularly upset and berated me for quitting the UK and so giving up my chances of achieving distinction in my profession by holding one or more of the highest offices in dentistry. I told him that I was tired of holding offices in which, due to circumstances beyond my control, I felt impotent, and that I wanted to do something more satisfying before I retired. Having spent most of his professional life developing the Newcastle Dental School from virtually nothing to be the largest provincial school in the UK this struck a chord with him and we remained firm friends for the rest of his life. I have never regretted this change in the direction of my life and am glad that I made it.

## Chapter Eight

# Hong Kong

Hong Kong in 1978 was an exciting place to live and work, it literally hummed with activity and all kinds of major developments were in progress. I loved being part of it for the six years that I lived there despite the unimaginable happenings in the last two years which I describe later. Due to the success of the localisation policy most of the key posts were held by able and well educated Chinese and the expatriate population was small being largely composed of those, like me, who had specific knowledge or skills not available locally and were thus a most interesting group of people, engaged in all kinds of activities ranging from building the underground railway under the tenement buildings in Victoria and Kowloon to piloting Jumbo jets. There was an excellent relationship with their Chinese counterparts who dominated the commercial and trans-hipment activities and the trades related to diamonds and other precious stones.

I left Britain where most of my colleagues and friends were firmly convinced that the targets set for the dental project by the Hong Kong Government were unrealistic and unattainable. They would probably have been right if my challenge had been located in the UK but having savoured the atmosphere in Hong Kong on a number of occasions during the previous two years I was convinced that it could be successfully completed on time there. In the event it was, but not before many problems, some of them completely unforeseen, had been overcome. During the previous two decades I had spent a great deal of time thinking about and discussing dental education and had been concerned in one capacity or another with building developments in the dental schools in Newcastle and Cardiff as well as those in Guy's and the Royal. I was convinced that the future of dentistry lay in both the preventative approach to the dental diseases and the dental team approach to established disease. I was only too well aware of the fact that my views were an anathema to my more conservative colleagues in dental academia but was encouraged by the enlightened attitude of the General Dental Council when they revised their guidelines for dental courses in the UK. In an attempt to ensure that the dental graduates from HKU were of an acceptable international standard one of the targets set by the HK Government was that the BDS (HK) degree be accepted by the GDC for registration purposes in the UK from its inception – quite a challenge! I was also only too well aware that even if my academic colleagues in the UK had accepted my views the constraints imposed by both the buildings in which they operated and the facilities available to them would have rendered the introduction of courses based upon them a virtual impossibility. The HK Dental Project offered me the opportunity to plan the buildings and facilities in which to introduce courses in line with my views. I felt that the high cost of dental care made it necessary to try to reduce the incidence of dental disease as much as was possible and to delegate routine items of dental care to ancillary workers wherever this was practicable in a similar way to that employed in medical practice. The implications of such practices made it necessary to train all members of the dental team in one institution and to train the leader of the team, the qualified dental surgeon, in management skills. I felt that these approaches were particularly appropriate for a developing country in which the overall standards of practice left much to be desired and unqualified illegal dentists still practised in the 'walled city' in the New Territories.

I was especially fortunate in that the Chief Dental Officer of Hong Kong, Dr Jim Yap, was a member of the Dental Academic Advisory Committee and, sharing my vision, he prepared room schedules for a dental hospital and school capable of meeting my objectives which were endorsed by both the DAAC and the HKU PGC and accepted by the HK government. It was also my good fortune that YRM International were appointed as architects, and Ove Arup and Partners as engineers for the Dental Project. The design team was led by a delightful South African architect, John Ross, who was both imaginative and outstandingly talented. He had played a key role in building the new St Thomas's hospital when I was on the staff there but we had never met prior to being involved in the HK Dental Project. It was a joy to work with him for, unlike some of his colleagues, he listened patiently to the views of the potential users and did his utmost to meet all their requirements. In my view the resulting building was a masterpiece and a monument to his skills and ability. As the room schedules were being discussed in the DAAC it became obvious that because of my specialist surgical background the detailed design and equipment schedules of both the dental laboratories and the non surgical clinical facilities were beyond me as I, and indeed all other members of the DAAC, lacked the necessary expertise. Thus it was decided to support the Dean, when appointed, by advertising a Chair in Conservative Dentistry and the post of Chief Technician Instructor.

Dr C.E. Renson, a Reader in the London Hospital Medical College Dental School at which he had participated in Government funded experiments in surgery design was appointed to the Chair. Mr Barry Shaw, the Chief Technician Instructor in the new Leeds Dental School who had played a key role in planning and developing the dental laboratories there was appointed to the other post. Together we drew up lists of design features for the architects and engineers and the equipment schedules required by the University for tendering purposes. We also suggested to HKU that the tender should be of the 'turnkey' type in which one supplier supplies everything rather than involving a host of suppliers. HKU accepted this suggestion as they agreed that it should minimise complications and facilitate the project, and went out to tender on this basis. The Secretary to the DAAC was a Registrar in HKU, Peter Walker, a delightful and able British emigrant to Australia and I arranged for him to have secretarial assistance from the British Dental Association during his visits to London.

During the months in which I was working my notice at the Royal he came to London bearing the bids for the equipment contract and a request from HKU for a report on each of them. Ted Renson and I, who were still fully employed in the University of London, met up with Peter whenever it was practicable to do so, usually in the evenings and at weekends. We were very concerned to discover that no bid was complete, some being very limited, thus making it difficult if not impossible to make a meaningful comparison between them. After discussion we decided to restrict our report to those tenders capable of fulfilling the 'turnkey' requirement in principle if not in full. As no two of these covered exactly the same list of equipment we drew up a schedule of key items to use for comparison purposes. Not surprisingly no dental supplier in Hong Kong had been able to submit a meaningful bid and all those that we had agreed to consider came from locations far away from the Colony. We decided that repairs, maintenance and the supply of spare parts could be a problem because of distance and that we should only recommend the purchase of items of equipment which had proved to be 'student proof' either in our own or another UK school. Peter Walker drew up a document detailing these procedural guidelines together with the thinking behind them and obtained HKU's blessing for us to use them. This we did and we began the mammoth task of preparing a detailed report on the various tenders. It emerged from our endeavours that only two of the tenders appeared to meet many if not all of HKU's requirements and that clarification of certain details of these was desirable. After getting permission to do so we invited representatives of the two companies involved to meet us on separate occasions in order to discuss and clarify these matters and did so as soon as it was practicable. This took a little time to organise and we finished our deliberations only a few days before our report was required in HKU. Worse still, Ted Renson was due to fly to the USA the next day and so we agreed all the points that we wished Peter Walker to include in the report and left him to draw it up as a matter of urgency.

One of the points was the relative size and reputation of the two suppliers one being a large well established and well known American company whilst the other was a small relatively unknown British company which had recently absorbed an even smaller company which it transpired had installed a number of dental chairs and units in the Royal, quite unknown to me, a few weeks or months earlier. When asked, Professor Keith Mortimer, the head of the department in which they had been installed was fulsome in his praise of both the equipment and the installation and we decided to mention his experience and views in the report. Peter worked very long hours preparing the report but it proved impossible to do so before Ted Renson flew to the USA. When it was complete I checked that its contents reflected our views accurately and signed it. Peter immediately flew back to Hong Kong with it leaving a copy for Ted Renson to sign on his return from America which he did. In the conclusion to the report we said that on the evidence before us we thought that the tender from Parkinson Bishop was overall the best but emphasised that we knew little or nothing of the company concerned and indeed were not competent to pass judgement on the manner in which it conducted its business. A day or two later the Tenders Committee met in HKU and awarded the contract to this small British company, and notified me of their decision before it was announced.

Soon after this I was shown two possible sites on which the hospital could be built. The larger of the two was flat and sited outside Victoria, the capital of the Colony, some distance from the University. A constant supply of suitable dental outpatients is an absolute necessity for effective dental teaching and I felt that this location would hamper and delay the process of building up a suitable clientele. The other site was in Sai Ying Pun bounded by Hospital Road and Eastern Street, a very busy area with excellent access for potential patients. Not only was it near to the University but it was adjacent to the Tung Wah Hospital, a non teaching general hospital which I felt had the capability of housing an Oral Surgery In-patient Unit and Day Bed Centre together with the potential for teaching medicine and surgery to dental students if facilities to do so were provided. Unfortunately the site was cramped and housed the Sai Ying Pun Jockey Club Clinic which would have to be demolished if the Dental Hospital and School was to be built there. The site also sloped steeply downwards to the north and a very high stone retaining wall had been built on its northern boundary so that it could be levelled when the clinic was built. Because the rock base was unstable and there was a history of tower blocks nearby having moved and collapsed during typhoons, extensive groundwork designed to produce a stable base on which to erect such a large and complex building would have to be undertaken.

After detailed discussions with the consultant architects and engineers I recommended that the Sai Ying Pun site be chosen and both the Government and the University accepted my advice. At that time I was delighted at the speed of decision making which was in sharp contrast to my experiences in the UK and augured well for the project. Little did I know how such events and one's motives could, and would be distorted by others for ulterior reasons to my detriment later.

In addition to the room schedules it had also been necessary to draw up a new dental curriculum. Fortunately the enlightened recommendations of the General Dental Council in the UK facilitated this process. Together with those academic staff who had been recruited but had not yet taken up their posts I produced a curriculum for a course in which the basic medical sciences and the clinical sciences were integrated to the benefit of both and teaching was predominantly on a small group basis. We chose groups of eight students for most activities but in some instances planned practical teaching on a half group basis and designed facilities such as phantom head laboratories to facilitate this. We believed in the team concept of clinical dentistry and made arrangements for the various types of team members to be trained under one roof. The only exception to this was the training of dental technicians which for various reasons had to be undertaken elsewhere. There was a small dental technology school in the Hong Kong Polytechnic which was situated in Kowloon which, with our assistance, was later upgraded to provide the standard of training required. Barry Shaw played a key role in this exercise which was a resounding success.

I spent many hours explaining the views, desires and requests of the Academic staff to the Consultant architects and engineers who listened patiently and long before attempting to translate them into customised physical facilities. This they did brilliantly and the resultant hospital offered facilities for dental research and education which at the time were considered to be second to none anywhere in the world. The building was designed to minimise the number of persons travelling in a vertical direction, clinical departments with the largest patient attendance being sited on the lowest floors and administrative offices, the library, research laboratories etc on the upper floors. The building was constructed on a modular principle and provided access for physically handicapped patients either in wheelchairs or on trolleys to all departments. The clinical departments and units were colour coded in an endeavour to overcome the problems of language and literacy whilst all the capital dental equipment was standardised and of the same colour in order to minimise the number of spare parts held, maintenance and servicing. As the site was 100% occupied the possibility of expansion was catered for by providing 33,928 square feet of usable but unallocated space equipped with all main services on the fifth of the seven floors. This space is now occupied by the Data Processing Unit and the Speech Therapy School. The hospital has no Central Sterile Supply Department, sterilisation being undertaken on a departmental basis in order that all members of the dental team could be taught safe practices and how to maintain the instruments they use.

All of the 228 clinical positions were ergonomically designed to provide optimum conditions for the treatment of patients, either in the sitting up or lying down positions, by left handed or right handed operators working either in the seated or standing positions with or without ancillary assistance. 161 clinical positions were in open clinics, designed to afford patients the maximum amount of privacy whilst facilitating the supervision of student activities by academic staff. Services to each clinical position were standardised and catered for all the capital dental equipment used anywhere in the hospital. Those outlets which were not required in particular departments were capped off. This design feature provided the flexibility required to deal with future needs and requirements. The services were designed in such a way that the capital dental equipment in any clinical position can be taken out of commission for maintenance, repair or replacement without interfering with the services to any other workplaces.

The outstanding Oral Radiography Unit was supplemented by seven satellite radiation protected X-ray rooms in

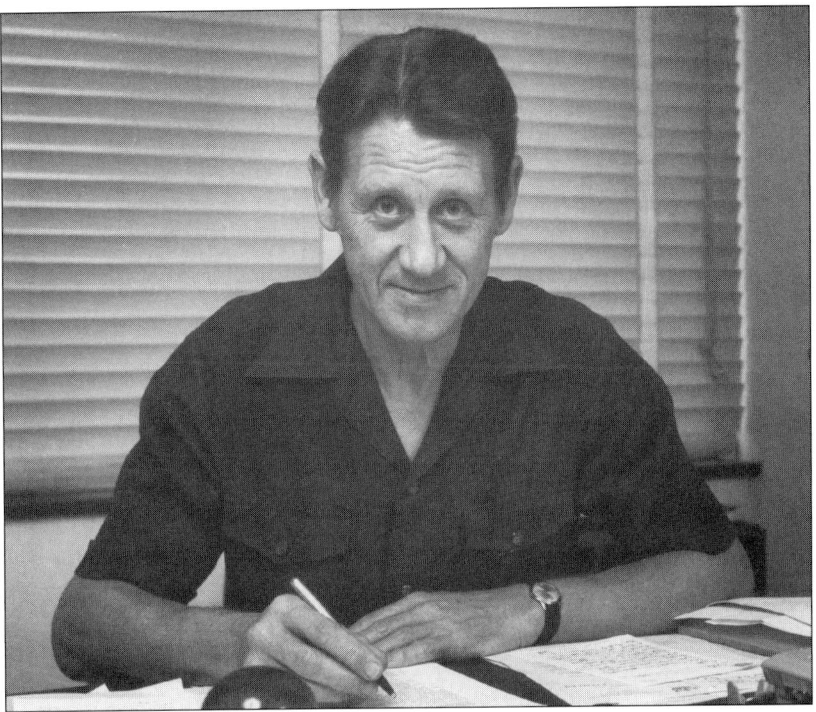

*At my desk in the Dean's Office of PPDH, Hong Kong.*

clinical areas each containing a dental X-ray machine and a daylight developer. The main facilities for dental technology were grouped together on the fourth floor adjacent to the Department of Prosthetic Dentistry and the Dental Materials Science Unit. Small satellite laboratories were provided in the other clinical departments. The two lecture theatres were exceptional acoustically and used primarily for the teaching of dental undergraduates and paradental trainees. They were sited in the Postgraduate Unit the services of which could be operated independently of the rest of the building thus facilitating out of hours use.

Offices for the academic staff were grouped together in the clinical departments in such a manner as to ensure privacy whilst permitting ready and quick access to treatment areas. A seminar room equipped with audio-visual aids was provided in each clinical department. The Dental Library occupied some 4130 square feet on the 6th floor. Seventy carrels were provided for private study and the library was kept open long after the hospital closed each day for the use of the many students needing a quiet place to study. Other features unique in dental hospitals at the time included an Oral Hygiene room in the Children's Dentistry Department where young patients received instruction in preventative dentistry and a resuscitation laboratory in which all types of students and staff in the hospital were taught to perform artificial respiration and cardiac massage. There was no fixed equipment in any of the surgeries in the Oral Surgery Out-Patient Unit, each of which was designed to provide staff access from both the front and the back of patients being treated by students all of whom were taught aseptic techniques. The OS seminar room could easily be converted to facilitate the teaching of basic surgical techniques on pigs' jaws before the students were allowed to treat patients. There were two large general anaesthetic operating theatres with both anaesthetic and scrub up rooms in which students were taught aseptic techniques and to operate on unconscious out patients. Some of the closed surgeries were equipped as phantom head rooms in which students were familiarised with all the capital equipment used in the clinics as distinct from that in the Main Phantom Head Room. A General Practice Unit was utilised to teach senior dental students whole mouth treatment planning and the differences between hospital and private practice.

The Prince Philip Dental hospital provides facilities for the treatment of out patients only. Eight day beds and sixteen in patient beds were provided for oral surgery in the nearby Tung Wah hospital in which the teaching of Medicine and Surgery was undertaken by members of the Departments of Medicine and Surgery of the University of Hong Kong. Although the unit was often hampered by the shortage of trained anaesthetists all forms of oral and maxillofacial surgery were undertaken in it often for the first time in the Colony. A thirty bedded oral surgery unit was designed which was built in the main teaching hospital, the Queen Mary Hospital after my departure from Hong Kong.

The initial hospital project was completed in less than five years from the start of the planning process, surely a record for such a complicated, massive and challenging undertaking. The Prince Philip Dental Hospital was officially opened by HRH the Duke of Edinburgh, Centenary President of the British Dental Association in March 1981. At that time it was only partially functional but in daily use. Success was achieved due to the exceptional efforts of many individuals too numerous to mention by name. There were many hiccoughs and hold ups en route and many changes of plan had to be made to cope with them. For one reason after another the building contractor failed to meet target dates for several stages of construction. The supplies department did not have proper storage space to house the medical and dental equipment when it was delivered and against all my protests it was literally dumped in a disused Army barracks totally unsuited for the purpose. Furthermore they made no arrangements to receive and check the first delivery and Ted Renson and I spent a very hectic weekend coping with this situation as best we could. The clinical facilities required to mount the first part of the integrated course were not ready on time and so we borrowed an unused government dental

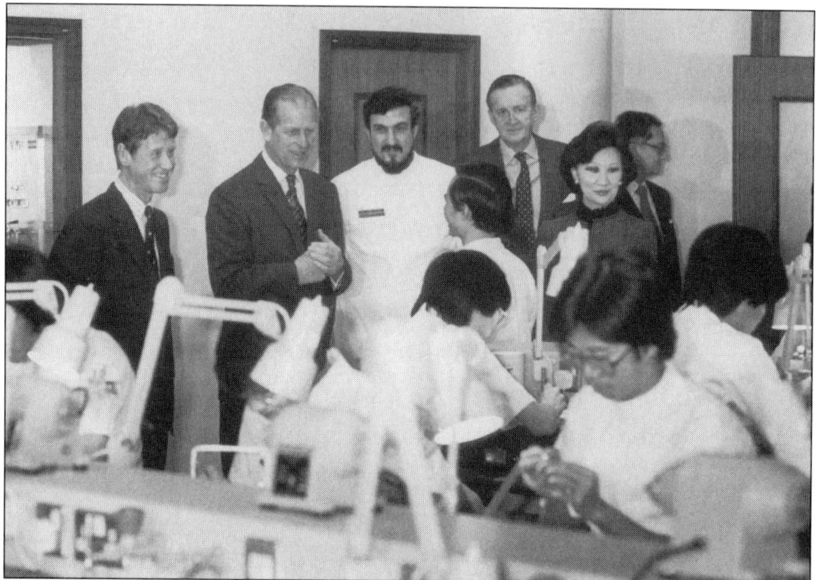

*HRH Prince Philip alongside Barry Shaw in the dental laboratory of PPDH. The Governor of Hong Kong, Sir (later Lord) Murray Maclehouse is next to the Hon (later Dame) Lydia Dunn.*

clinic which was awaiting either demolition or refurbishment, cleaned it up and installed some of the hospital equipment on a temporary basis so that the first intake of students could be admitted to the BDS course on the target date.

Whilst most Government officers were sympathetic, understanding and helpful some failed to understand either the complexity of the undertaking or the tightness of the schedule for completion imposed by the Hong Kong Government. Control of the finances of the Dental Project was vested in a special committee set up for the purpose and chaired by the then Deputy Financial Secretary, one Mr Henry Ching. He was unfortunately one such person and despite my being a member of the committee and giving good warning of when payments were due, on several occasions monies were not made available to meet our obligations. Finally, knowing the Governor, Sir Murray Maclehouse to be very supportive to the project, I sought an audience with him at which, accompanied by the Vice Chancellor, I explained the situation to him and warned him that if such difficulties continued there was little prospect of completing the Dental Project on time. He thanked me most courteously for being so honest and frank with him and took the necessary steps to resolve the situation. Needless to say my action did not endear me to the Civil Service in general and certain senior officers in particular who left me in no doubt as to their views. As I had realised when I took on the job of pushing the Dental Project through that it would not be a good basis for winning popularity contests I ignored the unpleasantness.

It was not only with civil servants and contractors that I had problems. There is, and always has been, a world shortage of first class dental academic staff and no dental school has a monopoly of them. Hong Kong University used the good offices of the Association of Commonwealth Universities based in London to recruit academic staff. This first class organisation used specially appointed independent expert assessors to prepare shortlists from the applications, interview suitable candidates and send a detailed written report containing their recommendations to the University who made the final decision in each instance. As Dean I played only a supporting role in this process by chairing the interviews and answering candidate's questions concerning Hong Kong, its University and the Dental Project. I did however have the power of veto when reports were considered by the University. With the benefit of hindsight I regret never having used this power and confining myself to expressing my reservations in certain instances for the appointees varied greatly in both performance and the way that they conducted themselves in office. A minority were exceptionally good, most were average and some, including one professor, were frankly failures who failed to meet their obligations on time and in full thus prejudicing the success of the entire project. I am afraid that this latter group found me a hard taskmaster as I was determined that the project would not fail because of their inadequacies.

Hong Kong at that time was a unique place in that it seemed to have the effect of magnifying the weaknesses of those who lived there. Thus if you liked a drink it was the easiest thing in the world to drink to excess or to become an alcoholic, if you smoked a little, to become a chain smoker, if you enjoyed socialising to become a complete hedonist, if you liked a flutter on the horses to become a compulsive gambler, if you were over confident, to become arrogant, opinionated and snobbish whilst if you were ambitious, to become ruthlessly so. Unfortunately there were examples of all these effects amongst the dental academic staff.

Once the hospital had been commissioned the Government set up a Board of Governors chaired by the Honourable Lydia Dunn OBE JP. She was a member of the Executive Council and had been most successful in the fashion industry. She had no experience in either Hospital or University administration and no experience whatsoever in medical or dental administration. She had an imperious manner and an excess of self confidence. Despite her inexperience in the field she made no attempt to learn from those who had and gave them little or no credit for their achievements when congratulated upon the success of the dental project to which she had contributed nothing. Her interference in the day to day running of the hospital which was my responsibility as Director caused friction between us and, as we failed to establish any rapport whatsoever, these were difficult days for me.

I loved living in Hong Kong, for although one was called upon to work long hours and extremely hard, there were many ways in which one could enjoy one's leisure. The climate for most of the year allowed one to swim once or more each day. There are many islands in the Colony and I had a fifth share in a pleasure junk which we used as a bathing platform off a number of them. A particular favourite was Lamma where every Sunday, after a walk over the peak and back, we used to indulge ourselves in a magnificent seafood meal in a Chinese restaurant built on a wooden platform above the shoreline which we called the Lamma Hilton.

I had a third share in a Pandora named *Pasisana*, my partners being a British Civil Engineer who worked for the HK Government and a delightful Chinese businessman who dealt in scientific apparatus. The Pandora was the smallest cabin class of sailing boat which raced regularly in the Royal Hong Kong Yacht Club. It slept four persons in acute discomfort but was usually used as a day boat. I had never raced before, having always been a cruising sailor in the UK and thoroughly enjoyed being instructed by my companions as we raced around the harbour every Saturday afternoon. Despite my ineptitude we had a considerable amount of success, especially in handicap races or heavy weather as the Pandora had a generous handicap and although small was an excellent craft in heavy seas. We also participated in Round the Island races and Regattas in both

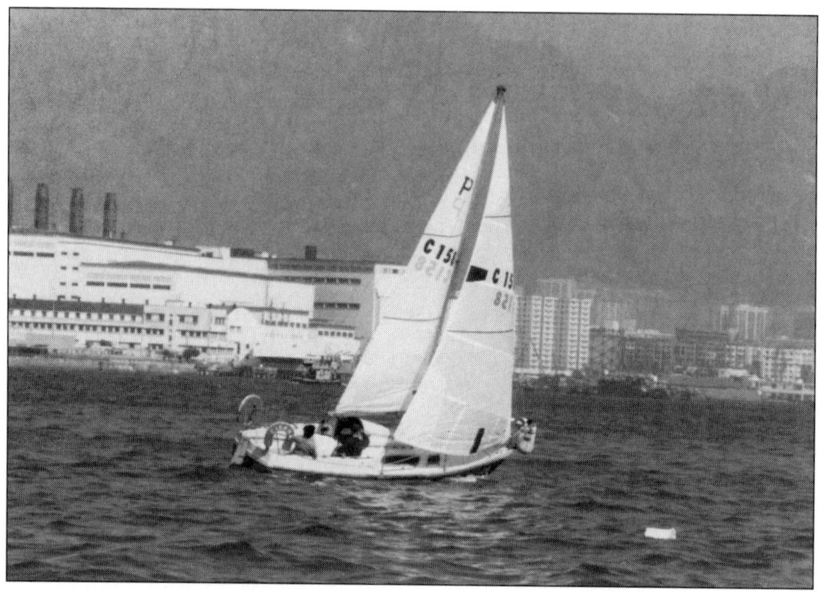

*Pasisana racing in Victoria Harbour.*

the New Territories and Aberdeen. It was a great delight to come into the splendid clubhouse, take a shower and drink beer and eat fish and chips out of newspaper on the balcony after the race. I enjoyed taking classes in the Yacht Club which enabled me to pass the Government examinations for Yacht Master and Engineer. Very sensibly no yacht is allowed to sail in the busy and crowded Victoria Harbour unless there is someone holding such qualifications aboard. After I obtained them I often took the boat out on my own in the evening after work.

In addition to the Yacht Club I was fortunate enough to be elected as a member of both the splendid Hong Kong Club and the United Services Club which was renowned for its Gurkha cuisine and relaxed atmosphere. I took lessons in Cantonese to the despair of my teachers and spent many happy hours alone with Heather walking on the various islands and in the New Territories. She loved butterflies and we spent many happy hours walking on Lantau Island where they outnumbered people many times. The Chinese love entertaining their friends in clubs and restaurants and we dined with them at least twice a week.

Life was good, the hospital was up and working well with few teething problems. The staff in the department had evolved into an excellent team who worked well together and the standard of oral and maxillofacial surgical care in Hong Kong had been transformed. The dental students were doing exceptionally well and impressing everyone with their enthusiasm, ability and industry. Most of us were very contented with our lot and then, without warning, everything changed.

In the beginning the equipment supplier performed well and both I and the university had only minor difficulties with them. However as the project progressed their performance began to deteriorate and I found myself in dispute with them over such matters as delayed delivery, unacceptable substitution of items etc. What I did not know at the time was that there was dissension between the directors of the company who were two couples. Apparently this came to a head and there was acrimonious litigation which resulted in one couple being required to forfeit both their directorships and their income from the Hong Kong dental project. Being aware that Hong Kong had some of the most draconian anti-corruption legislation anywhere in the world they resolved to use it to bankrupt the company. To this end they made a flying visit to the Colony during which they made allegations to the much feared Independent Commission Against Corruption (ICAC) that the HKU dental equipment contract had been secured by corrupt

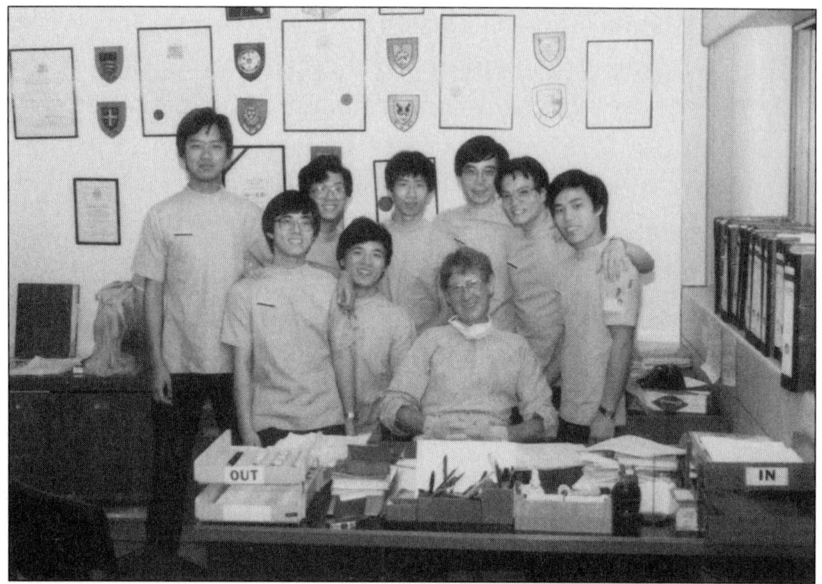


*With my first group of students in my departmental office in PPDH.*

means and left hurriedly. They were friendly with Ted Renson who had long been jealous of my success and lusted after my job as Dean and Director and he started making threatening telephone calls to me demanding that I resign in his favour or 'he would expose what Heather and I had been up to'! As I had not the remotest idea what he was talking about he got short shrift from me.

I now know that he denounced me to the ICAC as being corrupt and that under the then existing legislation they had no option but to investigate the matter fully. It may be said that he was misguided enough to believe that it was his duty as a citizen to take this action, however he went much further and aided by other dissident dental academia used the media to conduct a character assassination campaign against me. I was sitting in my office finalising details for a meeting of the Faculty Board to be held that evening when two ICAC officers burst in and insisted that I accompany them to their headquarters after arranging for all documents relating to the equipment contract to be made available to them.

In their offices I was astounded to learn of the allegations made against Messrs Parkinson Bishop and me for I could not believe that anyone in their right mind would take such allegations seriously. I told them that I had complete confidence in the integrity of my colleagues and did not believe that the dental project had been tainted by corruption. Furthermore, whilst the equipment suppliers had undoubtedly been guilty of some sharp practices, I had always found them straightforward to deal with. I recall that at the time I thought that the matter was just a storm in a teacup and so would soon be resolved. How wrong I was.

The first indication of my erroneous thinking was when I discovered that Heather was being interviewed in the next room having been 'picked up' during a simultaneous ICAC visit to our flat and she was even more surprised than I was by the experience. Having spent quite a bit of time in London whilst I was either in Hong Kong or travelling on University business she had acted as a point of contact with Paul and Brenda Bishop whom she had come to like and respect. They were Cockney sparrows who were superb ballroom dancers, having been World Latin American champions in spite of Brenda's considerable medical problems and disabilities. Despite having little or nothing in common with them we had had no difficulty in relating to them as the project progressed. I had served on the Dental Committee of the Medical Defence Union since its formation more than two decades before and had acted for them in the defence of members in Hong Kong and so become friendly with their solicitors in the Colony. As soon as we got home I contacted them and arranged to meet them the next day at which meeting they explained the horrors that awaited me despite my being completely innocent. How right they were for the investigations lasted for eighteen months during which I endeavoured to complete the project in the face of enormous difficulties caused by them.

One of my biggest problems was that I was prohibited by the draconian legislation from talking about any aspect of the enquiry to anyone other than my solicitor under threat of prosecution. Thus I was unable to defend my reputation as the character assassination attacks increased in both the University and the media. I felt like a criminal leper as colleagues fearful of compromising themselves shunned contact with me. I was not surprised to find that Lydia Dunn treated me like a criminal but was disappointed with the lack of support that I received from the Vice Chancellor, Dr Rayson Huang, with whom I had worked extremely closely and come to like and respect. I was disappointed to find that the attitudes of a number of my academic colleagues who should have known better was adversely affected by the scurrilous character assassination campaign. Despite all the rumours I was grateful to receive support from many others including the administrative staff in both the University and Faculty, including the University Secretary, Norman Gillanders and the Finance Officer, Graeme Large, and this enabled me to keep the project going forward albeit at a slower rate than planned.

I found solace in sailing, the company of true friends and walking on the islands with Heather. Time passed slowly and I must confess that I was at times both stressed and depressed, especially when contacted by friends in the UK and told that my reputation was being tarnished by the clumsy and heavy handed enquiries being conducted there by the ICAC. Thus I was relieved to be told that their enquiries were complete and the matter was closed despite there being neither a public announcement to this effect nor any apology for the damage done in the process, for mud sticks.

At the time I was serving as the President of the International Association of Oral Surgeons and in that capacity was invited to address the Annual Congress of the American Association of Oral Surgeons to be held in Atlanta, Georgia. The Academy of Dentistry International had also visited the Prince Philip Dental Hospital which they greatly admired and so had elected me to their Honorary Fellowship which was to be presented to me at their Annual Meeting in Las Vegas two weeks later. This meeting was to be held in conjunction with the annual meeting of the American Dental Association who had kindly elected me to Honorary membership. I decided to combine these official occasions with a holiday which both Heather and I sorely needed. We went once again to the 'Big Island' and Kauai in Hawaii before proceeding to Atlanta. Western Airlines lost our luggage en route and, as I was travelling in summer clothes, I had to borrow a suit, shirt, tie and shoes from an American friend and colleague, Andy Linz, to wear at the meeting.

After being reunited with our luggage we flew to New Orleans where we stayed with Bernice and Irving Sheen, old friends whom I had first met years earlier whilst giving a postgraduate course in the University there. This was fortunate for after a couple of days I developed abdominal pain and was admitted to the Ochsner Clinic with a ruptured appendix and peritonitis. For three or four days after surgery I was on intensive care. A week later I was discharged and convalesced in the Sheen home. Irving enlisted the help of my Oral Surgery colleagues in Las Vegas to permit me to spend a day or two at the meetings there before proceeding in a wheelchair/air journey to New York, and then on to London where I rested for a couple of weeks before flying to Hong Kong.

Unfortunately I arrived to find that in my absence the character assassins had stepped up their campaign to undermine confidence in me. Though far from fit I returned to work to find that the Vice Chancellor was very concerned about the situation in the Dental School and doubted whether I would be able to deal with it. Miss Lydia Dunn gave a sherry party to which all Heads of Department other than I were invited and my critics given open house to denigrate me. Colleagues were persuaded not to attend committees, making it impossible to proceed due to lack of a quorum. In these circumstances I felt that I had no option but to resign the Deanship and seek a mandate in the resultant election although I realised that this would be difficult as my critics had had a free rein to vent their spite for two years. However, once I had resigned I was heartened by the support that I received from colleagues who were sickened by what had gone on and who encouraged me to stick to my guns and sort out the mess.

Physically I was not strong enough to campaign actively but was led by my supporters to believe that I would be re-elected albeit by a small majority and not unanimously as previously. Quite obviously my opponents came to the same conclusion for they decided to split the anti-Renson vote. To this end one of my main supporters, Ian Davies, was persuaded to enter the contest at the last moment. His defection was a shock to me for, to put it kindly, administration and University politics were not his forte. Heather was especially hurt by his action as they had become very close friends both being gourmets and lovers of wine and music. He was single and they used to enjoy the special gourmet lunches after imbibing one or two 'bull shots' at the Peninsula Hotel every Saturday afternoon whilst I was racing around the harbour in *Pasisana.* Both were excellent cooks and used to delight in producing exquisite food for each other and their friends. Ian used to give most enjoyable dinner parties at which Heather supported him by acting as hostess.

In the event both Ted Renson and I lost and Ian Davies was elected as Dean. After a few days I resigned the Directorship of the hospital in his favour and for the rest of my time in Hong Kong I concentrated on running my department and developing oral and maxillofacial services in the Tung Wah and the Queen Mary hospitals. Morale and standards in the Prince Philip hospital declined even further as my opponents were able to influence affairs more and more. The retirement age in HKU was sixty but I had a gentleman's agreement with the Vice Chancellor that I would be extended for one year in order to see the first intake of dental students qualify. However, a combination of my changed circumstances and a marked deterioration in Heather's physical condition caused me to decide merely to honour the remaining fourteen months of my contract and not to apply for the promised extension.

It was not a happy time for me because I saw much that I had worked so hard for being thrown away, academic and clinical standards declining and good members of staff seeking pastures new. Having seen the harm caused by them

I regard character assassins as the garbage of society. They are usually inadequate people who are motivated by jealousy and greed, hardly the noblest of human qualities. These particular specimens cost Paul Bishop not only his business but also his marriage, me the Dean and Directorship, and dealt the Dental project a blow from which it has yet to recover. Despite these events Heather and I enjoyed our time in Hong Kong where we came to love the Chinese people and their industrious way of life, in particular my students who were so gifted and motivated as they struggled to pull themselves up by their shoelaces. They made all my years of hard work on the HK Dental Project eminently worthwhile and I am very proud of them. Even today almost two decades after these events I understand that one of the main character assassins seizes every opportunity that presents to bad mouth me. So be it, I despise and pity him.

Chapter Nine

# My First Retirement

Surprisingly perhaps, Heather had come through our dreadful ordeal in good spirits and not gone into depression over the unfairness of it all. She had long been aware of my complete lack of interest and expertise in money matters and had learned to cope with it. She was extremely astute and competent in such matters and had taken over the management of the family finances from the early days of our marriage to our mutual benefit. She had been opposed to my taking the appointment in Hong Kong until she was persuaded that the financial control of the Dental project was to be vested in a project finance committee chaired by the Deputy Financial Secretary and that I was to have no more financial responsibility than any other member of that committee. She knew that I had not been present at the committee meeting at which the award of the contract had been recommended and that the written opinions of the various tenders prepared by Ted Renson and me had been recorded by Peter Walker who had presented them to the Committee. Thus she could not understand how anyone could give credence to the false allegations made not against me alone but against both of us. However, she accepted the position and like me was sustained by the knowledge that as we had both given our all for the project and done nothing improper it was inevitable that we would be cleared of all charges. From her arrival in Hong Kong she had taken a personal interest in the housing provided for dental academic staff and their families, prepared for their arrival in the colony, especially when small children or babies were involved, often meeting them at the airport and providing food for the first day or two. When this process was complete she volunteered to work part time with a Chinese charity teaching handicapped children and found great happiness in this activity which she maintained throughout our stay in Hong Kong.

Physically, however, she was not doing so well and despite the medical care provided by the University Health Service was becoming progressively more disabled as her ability to walk was impaired. During our last year in Hong Kong she experienced severe back pain which was only partially controlled by analgesics. I decided to take her back to my old hospital, St Thomas', in which her life had been saved after

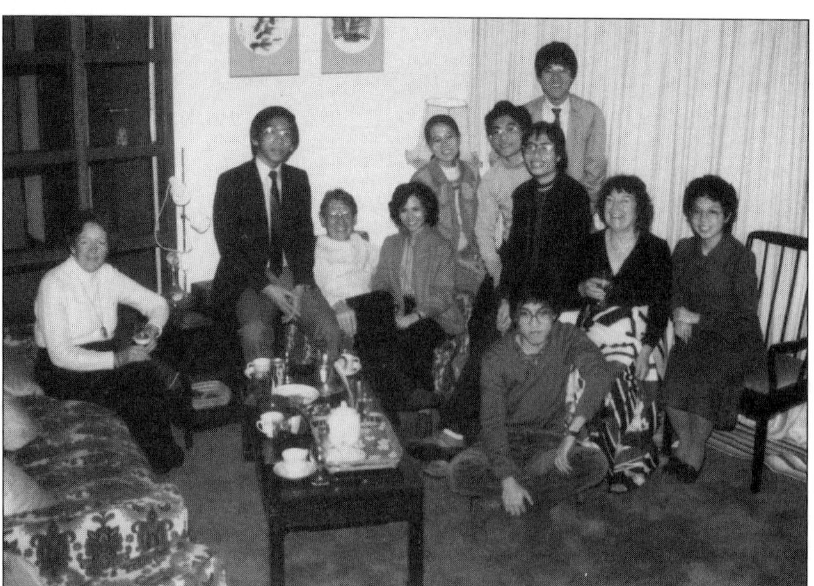

*Heather and I entertaining students in our flat.*

her accident, as soon as I had completed my contractual obligations to Hong Kong. She was opposed to this as she had become very attached to the first intake of dental students whom she regularly entertained and wanted us both to see them graduate. However, such was my concern for her that I insisted that we return to our home in South Croydon and seek the assistance of my former colleagues at St Thomas'.

They were absolutely first class and after extensive tests determined that her lumbar spinal canal was full of new bone, as a result of her injury, which was enclosing and pressing upon her cauda equina and four sets of lumbar nerves. Extensive spinal surgery was advised to resolve the situation and she was scheduled for early admission. Two or three weeks before Christmas we were told that a bed was available due to a cancellation. We took it and the operation was performed in Christmas week, technically all went well but she had a stormy post operative period in Intensive Care. She was leaking cerebro-spinal fluid and had a hypotensive crisis, a hypertensive crisis and a hypothermic crisis in quick succession. She later recalled that she awoke to find herself lying naked in a bed packed with ice and that the first person who spoke to her was a very black male nurse who had undoubtedly saved her life by cooling her in this way.

I spent the festive season visiting her whenever I was allowed to do so and praying for her recovery to a God I didn't believe in! Her condition slowly improved and after a week or two she was discharged to my care and I nursed her at home. She was very courageous and determined to walk again. More importantly she was no longer in severe pain and the pain that she was experiencing could be controlled with analgesics. She made excellent progress and whenever the winter weather permitted I encouraged and helped her to learn to walk once again. At first she could only manage a few steps with my support but as the days progressed she managed increasing distances without support. She was determined to shop in the Surrey Street Market, a famous open air market in central Croydon which she loved, and we rejoiced when she was able to do so once again. She set herself a series of targets and we achieved them one after the other as the weeks went by. Another of these was to have liver and bacon for lunch in the Crown and Sceptre, a splendid old pub at the bottom of the hill run by a delightful couple named Alan and Sally at the time. She was always keen on gardening and had very green fingers. I was, and am, exactly the opposite and can be guaranteed to pull up plants and retain weeds. In these circumstances she relished being a foreman directing a very unskilled labourer as we found happiness in bringing our neglected garden up to scratch. We bought a new music centre and television and began to visit and to entertain friends once again as the months progressed.

I have always loved my job and I missed the companionship of colleagues, the stimulation of students and the challenges of clinical work very much. Thus whilst I deemed it a privilege to care for Heather I cannot honestly say that I found it a fulfilling experience. She sensed this and as she felt guilty about my early retirement and believed that I still had something to contribute constantly urged me to find a new challenge. As her strength increased I began to consider doing this and made a few tentative enquiries.

About two years after her major surgery, in January 1987, I returned home from a meeting of the Representative

Board of the British Dental Association which I had attended in my capacity as a Vice President, to be told that she had accepted a job on my behalf earlier in the day. Professor Douglas Allen was a colleague and friend of mine from our days in Newcastle, whom I had not seen for at least two decades. He was, and is, a superb operator specialising in Restorative Dentistry and looked after Heather's teeth during our time in Newcastle. Being good looking and having a most attractive personality he was much admired by the fair sex and Heather was openly and unashamedly one of his principal admirers. Except for Christmas cards we had heard little or nothing from him since our ways had parted and so she had been surprised to receive a telephone call from him earlier in the day. In it he had told her that he was speaking from Jordan where he had accepted the challenge of setting up a new dental school under considerable difficulties. He was desperately in need of help, and having learned that I had retired from Hong Kong wondered if I would help him by spending a couple of months there teaching Oral Medicine. He knew nothing of Heather's medical problems and she did not enlighten him but said that I was available and would most certainly be pleased to help him in this way. In my day oral medicine did not exist as a separate speciality and I had always taught it in addition to oral surgery, local anaesthesia and the dental care of medically compromised patients. Although I knew nothing of Jordan or the Dental Project there I got out my lecture notes and other teaching aids and spent the next ten days in the BDA library preparing what I guessed would be a suitable two month course in oral medicine before flying out to Jordan, to be met by Douglas at the Queen Alia Airport near Amman.

Chapter Ten

# Jordan

NEVER HAVING BEEN to Jordan I was not familiar with its geography and it was a delight to find that the North of Jordan is very beautiful mountainous country and that parts of it are fertile enough to sustain two crops each year without the need for irrigation. As we drove north to Irbid, Douglas told me something of the country, its situation and the Dental Project before depositing me in the El Razi Hotel, then the sole establishment of its kind in Irbid. To say it was crummy would be generous for I arrived in February 1987 to find that the weather was very cold and I had brought only summer clothes, and that there was neither heating nor hot water in the hotel. Hardly an auspicious start, but I was tired after the journey and slept soundly despite the bed being uncomfortable and the shortage of bedclothes.

The next morning I was picked up and taken to the nearby Yarmouk University in which the Dental Project team was based. It comprised Douglas, one Jordanian, one Turk, one Egyptian and Henry Noble a distinguished dental academic from Glasgow who was giving a three month course in Oral Anatomy. All of the non British members of the team had obtained PhDs in the UK but had minimal clinical experience and no previous teaching experience. I learned that the first intake of dental students had been admitted to the University one year earlier despite there being no curriculum, staff, premises or clinical facilities available. They had spent the year being taught anatomy and physiology in the Faculty of Medicine by teachers who knew nothing of the essential needs of dental students. These studies had been supplemented by others in Arabic, English and Military Science and a course in the History of Medicine. Since his arrival a few months earlier Douglas had been striving to sort some kind of order out of the chaos but his efforts had been hampered by student riots in the University during which fatalities had occurred. The dental, medical, pharmacy and nursing students had not been directly involved in these troubles but the entire University had been closed for two months. Much of Yarmouk University was housed in temporary buildings pending completion of a new University campus near Ramtha a small town on the Syrian border about 20-25 kilometres from Irbid. Unfortunately work on this imaginative project had been suspended due to political and financial problems. However some buildings were either complete or almost so and the Government had decided to move the Engineering and Health Sciences Faculties into them from the Yarmouk campus to form a new institution, the Jordan University of Science and Technology (JUST).

When I arrived this process had just commenced and I was driven out into the desert to view the situation which was to say the least chaotic. The contrast with the carefully planned and staged early days of the Hong Kong Dental Project could not have been more stark. Furthermore Jordan was an extremely poor developing country devoid of oil revenues and housed more Palestinian refugees than citizens, many of whom still lived in refugee camps some forty years after leaving their homeland. I met my academic colleagues in all disciplines, many of whom were either refugees or the children of refugees, and the dozen or so dental students about half of whom were of Palestinian origin. Another surprise was to find that almost fifty per cent of them were women who were not taught separately from their male counterparts as in Saudi Arabia. They were a delightful group of young people, determined to pull themselves up by their shoestrings and to succeed despite all the problems. Their command of the English language was excellent and their intelligence soon apparent and I quickly became empathetic to them in their plight and felt that I wanted to help them as much as was practicable.

Certain things were immediately apparent to me, the first of which was that I had to get out of the El Razi Hotel. I was allocated a tiny flat in the Yarmouk campus in which Douglas and Henry were also housed together with other expatriates in all faculties. The flat was furnished but I had to buy towels, bed linen, cooking utensils, cutlery and crockery myself, using monies that I had brought with me. It was also obvious to me that the course in oral medicine that I had prepared was quite impracticable as the students had not studied pathology, bacteriology or general medicine and surgery and had never even examined each others' mouths. Douglas agreed with my assessment that I could be of more assistance to him in other ways and was particularly keen to draw on my experience as a Dean in the UK and Hong Kong as this was the first time that he had been in this position.

Despite the lapse of time since we had worked together in Newcastle we had always liked and respected each other and quickly established a working relationship. It soon emerged that I had not been sent a contract as I had to be vetted by security before I could be employed and so I was driven in a University car to Intelligence Headquarters in Amman to spend a long afternoon being questioned by a number of military officers on a variety of subjects including my academic career and military experience. Their manner was very gentlemanly and I was surprised to find that they were far more interested in the fact that I had been in Iran soon after the revolution acting in an advisory capacity for an International Agency than in my military service in Palestine or the several Israeli stamps in my passport. A few days later I was presented with a contract on a monthly basis whilst my academic credentials were verified. The salary offered was extremely low by UK or international standards but I was soon to learn that, because of my seniority, for I had been a Professor for twenty-eight years at that time, it was second only to that of the President of the University and more than covered the purchase of essentials there being little else to spend it on.

The President was a most impressive man being an endocrinologist of international standing who had trained and worked in both Germany and the United States and had served as Minister of Health prior to being selected by King Hussein to head the JUST project in which the monarch was particularly and passionately interested. The King was only too aware of the lack of natural resources in Jordan but wise enough to recognise that the culture and high intelligence of his people were his country's greatest asset. The Universities in Jordan were rapidly expanding in both size and number and produced the teachers, engineers and health professionals required by other less enlightened Arab countries. Such expatriates regenerated the Jordanian economy with their incomes. JUST was central to his plans

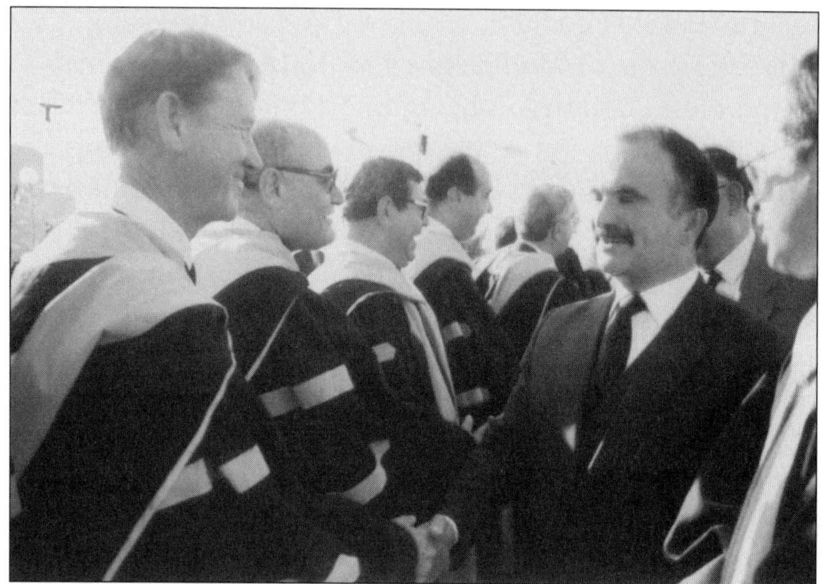

*The Deans meet Crown Prince Hassan during one of his regular visits to JUST.*

and he is said to have described it, when Dr Kamel Ajlouni had succeeded in establishing it on a sound basis, as the jewel in the Jordanian Universities' Crown. Dr Ajlouni was an inspirational, forthright, enthusiastic and energetic dynamo of a man who soon built up a most able team including Drs Faiz Kassouni and Mohammed Macusi, his Vice Presidents. The former was an agriculturist and the latter an electrical engineer and both had held senior academic posts in the United States. Later in the JUST project Dr Faiz was to found the Faculties of Agriculture and Veterinary Science before becoming the Governor in the Aqaba region where he stage managed the peace talks which were held there, after which he became the President of Yarmouk University.

Douglas asked me to first concentrate my efforts on producing a draft curriculum for dental studies and this I did, being ably assisted by the Faculty Administrator, Jamal Rousan, a Jordanian graduate in English in Cairo University who had held a similar post in Riyadh, Saudi Arabia, when the dental school was established there. The president had made it a policy that all JUST degrees would be of a recognised international standard whilst incorporating a number of components peculiar to Arab Universities. Jamal's guidance was particularly helpful to me in regard to these and our draft quickly gained acceptance with minor modifications by Douglas, the Presidency and the Dean's Council and was submitted to the Government for approval. The buildings on the JUST site had been designed for other purposes and were completely unfurnished when we first took them over. Teaching went on whilst seating, blackboards, screens etc. were installed and of necessity much of it was of an informal nature which resulted in a close bonding between members of the Academic staff and their students. A dental mechanical and a pre-clinical phantom head laboratory were set up in which the students were instructed in basic practical techniques. Palestinian colleagues in the Medical Faculty consulted us about the requirements of our students and produced excellent courses in anatomy, physiology, pharmacology, pathology, medicine and surgery.

The isolation of the JUST campus made it an unsuitable site for clinical teaching which is entirely dependent upon the attendance of adequate numbers of suitable outpatients. When the Medical Faculty moved to the JUST site they continued to provide a health service on the Yarmouk campus and maintained an out-patients clinic in Irbid for this purpose. The top two floors of this building were vacated by the nursing faculty and were converted, not without difficulty and delay, into a Dental Clinic with twelve clinical workplaces and supporting facilities. As treatment was provided free we were swamped with patients, many of them totally unsuitable for the needs of teaching. It was a difficult situation as we had to be highly selective and turn many members of the staff of both Universities and their families away despite them being eligible for treatment under the provisions of the University Health Service. Much ill will was engendered until they became persuaded that the Dental Clinic was funded purely for teaching purposes and not as part of the Health Service.

I supervised the setting up of the clinical facilities which took almost a year whilst Douglas concentrated on the recruitment of both teachers and ancillary staff such as dental technicians and dental surgery assistants. We had one excellent Jordanian dental technician, Ismael Nawasra, who spoke excellent English and had worked with expatriate dentists in Saudi Arabia for some time and so was familiar with modern techniques. He played a key role in the development of dental laboratory services. His wife was an English dental surgery assistant who helped us when the needs of her very young family permitted her to do so. Douglas decided to set up a training course for dental surgery assistants and recruited four British DSAs as teachers on it. Both of us spent many hours in small group teaching of the dental students and became very attached to them. Douglas also dealt personally with almost every aspect of the complex running of the Faculty and in consultation with the Presidency and the Dean's Council prepared draft regulations for the Faculty. Both of us tried desperately to recruit colleagues in all the dental disciplines so that we could implement the curriculum. In this we were only partially successful for we had little to offer other than challenges and both pay and conditions compared very unfavourably with those offered by the surrounding oil rich states. The calibre of many of the recruits, especially those who had trained in Egypt and never worked anywhere else, was unsatisfactory and there was a continuous turnover of staff. At that time all Jordanian dentists had trained abroad in countries all over the world as diverse as Yugoslavia, India, the Philippines and Bolivia in addition to Egypt, Turkey and Iraq. Few if any of them had any specialist academic qualifications or experience. JUST recruited a number of them to assist us with a view to sending the best of them on scholarships to the UK and the USA for postgraduate training at a later date. With the active encouragement of the Medical Faculty I set up a very basic oral and maxillofacial surgery service in the Princess Basma Hospital in Irbid and began to operate there despite grave deficiencies in both anaesthetic and nursing services.

It was not all work, for in this strictly Sunni Muslim society the University was closed on Thursdays and Fridays. Douglas had a splendid old Mercedes and every weekend we used it to explore and picnic in different sites in Jordan which is an archaeological treasure trove. I was and am particularly fond of Um Queis, the biblical city of Gadara of the Gadarine Swine. Its remains surmount a hill which overlooks the Golan Heights and Lake Tiberias (Sea of Galilee). This wonderful place is only about twenty kilometres from Irbid by the direct route and we often went there returning via the Jordan valley. Another favourite of mine is Jerash which is about twenty-five miles south of Irbid and full of Roman artefacts although only partially excavated. The grooves cut by chariot wheels in the cobblestones are clearly visible as are the drains under the streets which still work. The streets in Irbid, a dusty Arab town, do not have drains and become flooded and break up in rainy weather. The motorway which now connects Irbid to Amman was then in the early stages of construction and we used to drive down a winding narrow road with spectacular mountain views lined by mimosa trees in blossom and six foot high wild hollyhocks in season. As government employees we could stay at the Amra Hotel for a modest charge and use its splendid pool which was one of the few places in which mixed bathing was permitted other than in Aqaba.

Time passed quickly and both our wives enjoyed holidays with us during this period in which the Dental Project progressed rapidly. Unfortunately Douglas's wife Brenda was a severe asthmatic and was the victim of an attempted rape whilst resting alone in his flat and his car was damaged at the behest of an unsatisfactory employee whom he had dismissed. Both of them became disillusioned with the project and Douglas decided not to renew his annual contract. At this time I was still on monthly contracts and I accepted his invitation to drive home with him in his car. When it became known that I intended to leave I came under great pressure from the Presidency and others to stay on and to succeed Douglas as Dean. However it was only when the dental students as a group pleaded with me to stay on so that they would have the chance to qualify that I agreed to do so.

I bought myself a thirteen year old Mercedes which ran beautifully and was undoubtedly the best car that I have ever owned and which enabled me to do the job. I pulled out all the stops to recruit academic colleagues and was absolutely

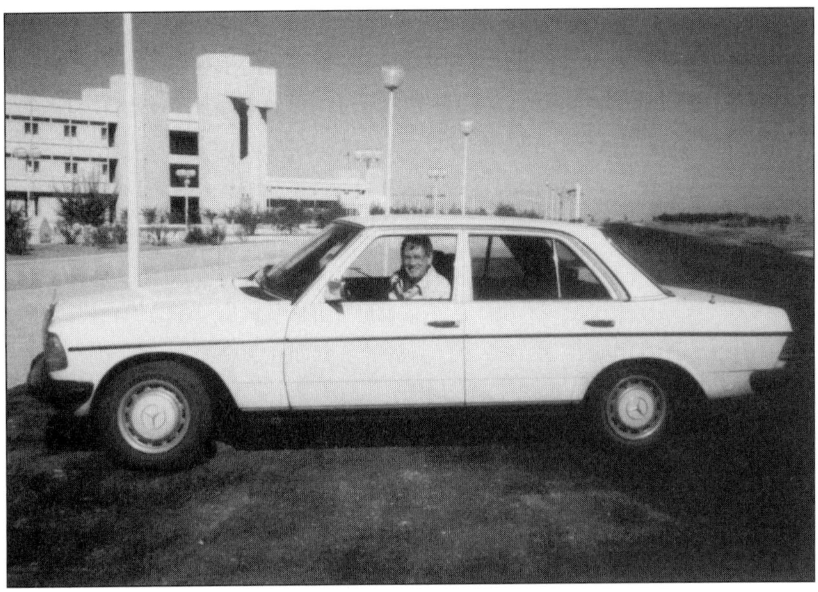

*Me in my ancient but much loved Mercedes in JUST.*

delighted when Geoff Shaw replaced Douglas as Professor of Conservative Dentistry for although we had never worked together I was well aware of both his abilities and personal qualities from my time as an external examiner in Birmingham.

Another acquisition was Duncan Macmillan as Professor of Prosthetics. We had worked together in both Newcastle and Hong Kong and so I knew that he would be a great success in Jordan and he certainly was. His Canadian wife, another Brenda, had been Senior Tutor in the DSA school in Hong Kong but readily agreed to serve under Yvonne Patience, an Australian who had been her junior in Hong Kong, and who had taken up the post of Senior Tutor in Jordan a couple of months earlier. Together they really improved the standards of DSA training and when Yvonne left, for family reasons, a year or so later, Brenda took over from her. Geoff Shaw was joined by a Polish Professor, Honorata Limonowska, whom he later married. When he finally retired they moved to Poznan where Honorata is now Dean of Medicine. The Dental Faculty at this time was known as the League of Nations for it had twelve members from eight countries including Iraq, Egypt and India.

These were happy times for although we worked long hours we enjoyed many social activities with both the students and each other and were delighted with the way that both our young Jordanian and Palestinian colleagues and the students progressed. In order to ensure standards I persuaded the University to employ External Examiners from the UK at each stage of the course. Although we could offer them little, no one invited to serve declined and invariably expressed their surprise and delight at the standards achieved by the students. All was going well when Faiz Khasouni, who was Acting President at the time, showed me a sheaf of newspaper cuttings detailing the problems that I had experienced in Hong Kong which had been sent to him anonymously. With a broad smile he said that he had read them all and wished to congratulate me on the way that I had behaved in a difficult situation. He then binned them.

The first intake of dental students all graduated at first attempt, several of them with honours, and received their degrees from King Hussein in a splendid open air congregation with bands playing and flags flying and the staff in academic dress. It was joy to see their families, some Bedouin, others Palestinian refugees, excitedly applauding them, as individually they shook hands with their King as he congratulated them on their success. We selected the six best of them to work in the Dental Clinic in preparation for an

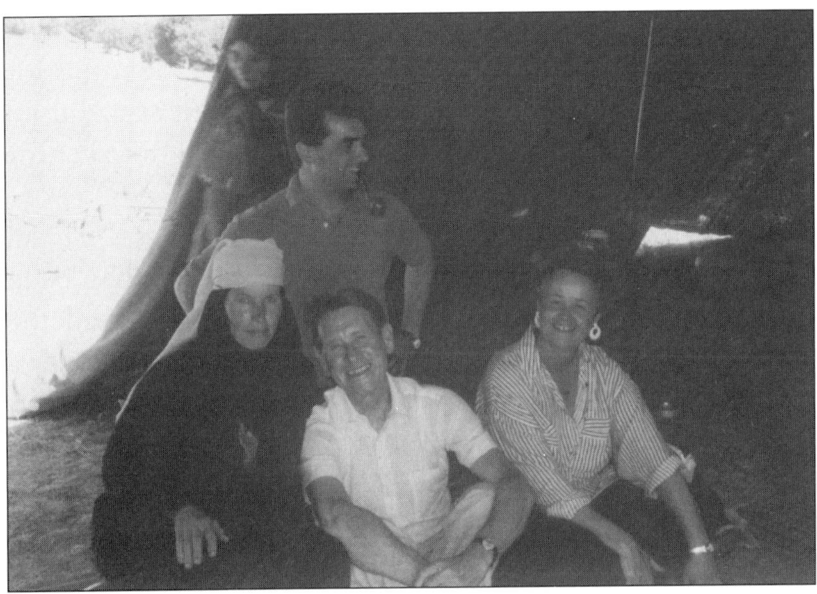

*Brenda McMillan and I visiting friends in a Bedouin tent.*

academic career. All of them later went to the UK on scholarships and obtained either the FDS diploma or a PhD degree or both making an excellent impression on their British senior colleagues as they did so.

The Gulf War erupted and both British and American flags were burned in the streets of Amman. Refugees of many nationalities streamed into Jordan from Kuwait. The authorities coped with the situation very well and many of them were repatriated during the next few weeks. Feelings ran high, especially so in the Palestinian refugee camps in which there was great support for Saddam Hussein. In the midst of this I and those of my colleagues who remained continued to carry out our duties without any problems. All the locals appreciated what we were doing there, were grateful to us and treated us with respect. In the midst of this chaos I received the news that Heather had suffered a severe relapse and was very unwell. At the time it was almost impossible to leave Jordan as there were many applicants for every plane seat. Only after the Acting President had used his good offices for a week did he obtain a flight ticket for me and I flew home.

When I arrived I found Heather in severe pain having had a recurrence of her lumbar spine problems. She had been seen by the consultant surgeon who had performed the major spinal surgery on her and was on the waiting list for a repeat performance. It was soon obvious to me that her agony was not being relieved effectively by the plethora of drugs that she was taking and I sought means to expedite her admission. Fortunately I had taken out private medical insurance for her after she recovered from her previous major surgery and so she was admitted to a private hospital in which the same surgeon operated upon her back once again. Whilst the operation went as planned and she stood it well she never again had normal sensation below the waist nor proper control over her natural functions. Despite this she was determined to live as normal a life as possible and courageously overcame her disabilities, hiding them from others. Although she could not feel her feet she learned to walk again with my assistance and dealt with her other problems with a quiet dignity that one could not help but admire.

Some years earlier we had bought a small beach side villa adjacent to Sabinillas, a small fishing village in the Costa del Sol. As is usual the developer had gone bankrupt and we had many problems with it. During my four year stint in Jordan it had stood forlorn and empty. At Heather's behest I flew out to Spain and camped in it whilst builders repaired, upgraded and decorated it and after a couple of months was able to take her there to convalesce. She always loved living in the sunshine in such beautiful surroundings and her condition improved rapidly. We returned to Croydon and enjoyed a quiet life in our home and garden.

In the meantime, Geoff Shaw had taken office as Dean and carried the project forwards. JUST was kind enough to invite me to act as an external examiner and during a ten day visit I could see that things were progressing well as some of our Jordanian colleagues were returning having completed their postgraduate studies. At the time of my visit Geoff told me that he had been offered a much better paid appointment in Saudi Arabia which he was considering accepting. Having been there I pointed out that life and work in Saudi would be very different from that he had experienced in Jordan and I was saddened when some weeks later I learned that he had decided to leave JUST. About a year later I started receiving telephone calls from Dr Saad Hijazi, who had been Dean of the Faculty of Medicine in my day but had been promoted to Vice President of the University. In essence he told me that the Dental Faculty was in crisis and asked me, on behalf of Dr Ajlouni to go back to Jordan and sort things out. I explained Heather's condition to him and told him that regretfully I was not in a position to help JUST. Heather was very upset when she learned of this conversation for through letters from Jordanian friends she was more aware of the situation in the Dental Faculty in JUST than I was and knew that many folk there hoped that I would help to resolve the problems. During the next two or three months she made a determined effort to demonstrate to me that despite her disabilities she could cope on her own and was keen to do so if I was invited again to help.

I was asked again a few months later and I agreed to fly

out to Jordan and review the situation in the Dental Faculty in order to see if there was anything that I could do to improve the situation. My dental colleagues were not told of the date and time of my arrival and I was met by a University driver on his own, who was fortunately an old friend, and after several phone calls was deposited in the El Razi Hotel once again for the weekend. News travels fast in such societies and I was delighted to be visited there by some of my former students who were especially dear to me. From them I learned something of their problems and the reasons why morale in the Dental Faculty had collapsed. My concern increased when on the Saturday I was told bluntly by Dr Ajlouni, the President, that he was ashamed of the Faculty and intended to shut it down unless I could get it functioning properly again. He provided me with an office in the Presidency and the services of Jamal Rousan on a half time basis.

It was soon apparent to me that things had started to go wrong almost as soon as Geoff Shaw had given up the Deanship. A very junior Palestinian colleague who had been working in Kuwait but had no academic experience whatsoever, had been made the Dean. He needed all the support and guidance he could get but instead of providing it Dr Hijazi, the Vice President responsible for the Faculty had moved Jamal Rousan to the Presidency to help him deal with international affairs. Several experienced expatriate teachers had left and those who remained, like Professors Nestor Hollist and Kamala Pillai, were sidelined as feuding between Jordanian and Palestinian teachers grew. Student numbers were increased and funding provided for an extension to the clinic which was partially built. Even a cursory examination revealed both defects and deficiencies in it and that those responsible for it had little or no idea of what they were doing. The young colleagues who had completed their post graduate studies overseas were returning to a dental school in chaos bedevilled by factional rivalries.

The administration of the Faculty itself was chaotic and although the Dean, whose contract had been terminated was still in JUST there was no handover/takeover and I never met him during my second tour of duty in the University. Against strong opposition I recommended to the Presidency that the Heads of the two Departments and the Director of the Clinic, all annual appointments, continue in office for a further year. I reconstituted the Faculty Board in accordance with University statutes and acted as its Secretary in addition to being its Chairman thus ensuring that it functioned properly once again. The responsibilities of all individual members of the staff of the Faculty were determined and clearly defined and a number of matters of dispute resolved. The clinic extension was extensively re-designed before building recommenced and programmes for equipping it, commissioning it and operating it were drawn up. Each local member of staff was interviewed individually and a programme for their professional development suggested. As morale in the Faculty improved, weekly seminars were held at which individual teachers presented details of research that they either had or were conducting and these talks were usually followed by a lively discussion. A number of experienced Iraqi teachers, who had been working elsewhere as expatriates, were recruited and the situation stabilised and so the Faculty began to go forwards once again. There were dramatic improvements in both clinical and academic standards both in the Faculty and especially so

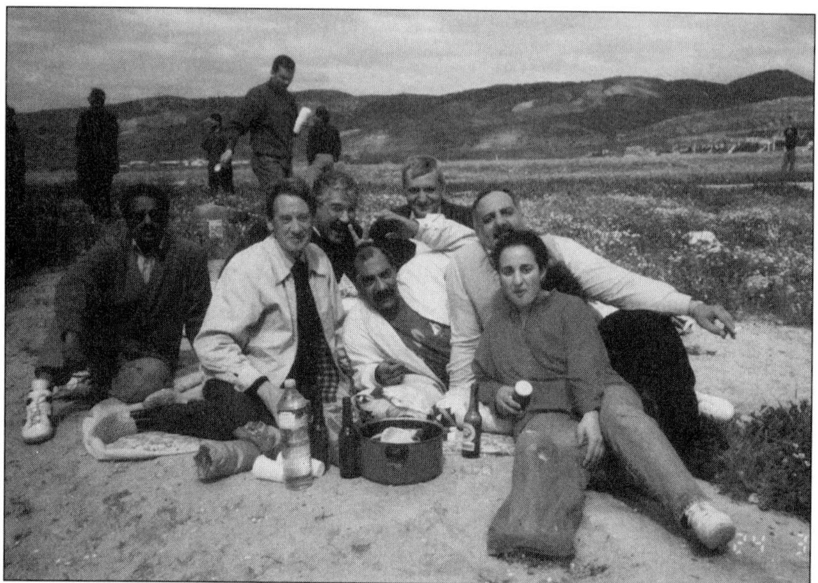

*A staff picnic. Dr Anwar Bataineh is on my left with his arm raised.*

in the oral and maxillofacial surgery service once Dr Anwar Bataineh had returned from his postgraduate studies in Leeds. The year passed quickly and was crowned by the favourable comments of the External Examiners.

As there was still much to be done if these achievements were to be consolidated I agreed to stay on for another year. New Heads of Department and a new Director of the Dental Clinic were appointed and the localisation scheme for academic staff regenerated. To this end a Primary FDS course was instituted with the enthusiastic support and co-operation of teachers in the basic medical sciences in the Faculty of Medicine. The course was held during evenings and weekends and lasted for a year. It was free to Clinical Dental Officers working in the Clinic and open to all other dental colleagues at a nominal fee. At the end of the course JUST hosted a Primary FFD Examination held by the Royal

College of Surgeons in Ireland. Six of the nine entrants from JUST passed the examination at this their first attempt, a remarkable achievement, and the examiners were kind enough to say that the standard of the candidates overall was exceptional in their experience. Postgraduate places were obtained in British Universities for over a dozen scholars from JUST during the year and scholarships awarded. The Faculty held a most successful two day Open Scientific Meeting, with the aid of a grant from the British Council, at which staff, students and visiting colleagues made presentations. The Minister of Health, a doctor, and many other dignitaries attended the meeting and were favourably impressed by the contributions of the younger members of staff and the students in particular.

At the end of the year Dr Ajlouni retired from the Presidency and was replaced by Dr Saad Hijazi. Nice man though he is, Dr Saad's appointment was of concern to me for, in my view, he was largely responsible for the state of the Faculty which had occasioned my return to Jordan. Like many other medical academics he had never either understood nor appreciated the especial problems of dental education and he resented its expense. The essential nature of the practical vocational training involved have rightly earned dental education the sobriquet of the cuckoo in the University nest! The high cost of both the equipment and materials used and the high staff:student ratios required for the essential protection of patients allowing themselves to be treated by learners combine to create this situation. There was no malice in Dr Saad's actions, which in my view were entirely due to a lack of appreciation of essential relevant factors, but I feared for the future of the Faculty under his Presidency.

In an attempt to ensure that the essential needs of the Faculty were not overlooked I agreed to stay on for yet another year. This proved to be my most difficult year in Jordan during which all my fears were realised. The JUST success rate in the Primary FFD examinations increased and excellent custom-made postgraduate places were obtained in the UK for a record number of potential dental academic staff but no scholarships were awarded. Against my advice it was decided to introduce private practice into the Dental Clinic causing a marked decrease in the clinical experience of the students due to the limited clinical facilities. This problem was compounded by an increase in the number of dental students and the introduction of degree courses for both dental technicians and chairside ancillary workers. The final straw came when less that three months after publicly telling three long serving and excellent expatriate teachers that JUST required their services for another five years at least, Dr Saad terminated their contracts. He did this whilst I was in the UK on compassionate grounds as Heather's condition was causing concern. On my return to Jordan it was obvious to me that there was a complete breakdown of understanding between the President and myself and so I completed the two months left on my contract and returned home to look after Heather. Except for liaising with my Jordanian postgraduates in the UK and commenting on, and sometimes re-writing scientific papers for my colleagues in the Medical and Dental Faculties in JUST that was effectively the end of my academic career. At the age of seventy-two I had had a good innings and so retired once again for the third and final time.

Chapter Eleven

# Dental Politics

I entered the dental political arena by chance when my name was literally pulled out of a hat and I became the sole representative of the English provincial dental schools on the newly constituted Central Committee for Hospital Dental Services (CCHDS), an autonomous craft committee of the British Dental Association in 1964. During the succeeding years we battled with governments of both persuasions to preserve, maintain and improve the dental service of the NHS, open to all and free at moment of use. To my surprise I was elected, in my absence, to be the Vice Chairman of the Committee in 1970 serving under the Chairmanship of my long term friend and teacher, John Hovell. To my consternation it was then discovered that John had completed six years in that office and so was ineligible to continue in it and in this inauspicious way I became Chairman in his place in February 1971. I first learned of this situation when, in a telephone call from the Secretariat of the BDA I was asked to attend a meeting of the Representative Board of the BDA two or three days later at which the appointment of a new Association secretary was to be made. I knew nothing of either this matter nor the personalities involved and when the papers for the meeting arrived by courier I was surprised to learn that the candidate being put forward by the Selection Committee was not a member of the profession but a retired senior RAF officer named Alistair Mackie.

After reading his curriculum vitae I became convinced that, able as he might be, he was the wrong man for the job and I decided to oppose his appointment. I felt it only fair to telephone the Secretariat and notify them of my decision. It was suggested to me that I should see Ronnie Allen, the Vice Chairman of Council and Chairman of the Selection Committee, whom I had never met, before the meeting and I was informed that he would be spending the night before the meeting in a particular hotel but would be arriving there very late. I arrived at the hotel very early on the morning of the meeting and found him fast asleep having overslept. I introduced myself and stated the nature of my business and we discussed the matter whilst he quickly bathed and dressed. We agreed to disagree and entered the Board together late. It was the custom to introduce new members at their first attendance at a Board meeting and so the Chairman stopped the proceedings to extend this courtesy to me thus ensuring that everyone present knew who I was. The heated debate which had been in progress when we arrived then resumed and it soon became obvious to me that I was not alone in my reservations about the proposed appointment for a number of long serving members of the Board, including some Vice Presidents, made their opposition to the recommendation crystal clear. When called upon to speak I tried to present my views in a logical and non emotive way whilst making it very clear that I thought Mr Mackie's appointment would have disastrous consequences for both the Association and the profession it serves. To my dismay when it came to the vote Alistair Mackie was appointed for a probationary period. He had been waiting in the wings and was then introduced to the meeting. This was the first time I had seen him and my heart sank.

As Chairman of the CCHDS I was required to attend meetings of the Association's Council as an ex officio member. These were usually held monthly and I was saddened by the divisions on the Council which meant that minutes were constantly being challenged, the meetings were interminable and decisions, when made, were usually less than clear cut and almost inevitably too late. To make matters worse the new Secretary had failed to gain the trust and support of the administrative staff and was making ill considered attempts to impose what he believed to be 'modern management methods' on his juniors. The Chairman, George Gibb, and Vice Chairman faced almost insuperable difficulties in conducting the affairs of the Association and it was a very unhappy situation for everyone concerned. At my third Council meeting George Gibb announced his resignation as Chairman, having been appointed Chief Dental Officer at the Ministry of Health. At the meeting of the Representative Board which followed, only the second that I had attended, Ronnie Allen was elected as Chairman of Council and nominations for Vice Chairman called for. To my amazement, for I had not been consulted, I was proposed from the floor and quickly elected to office much to the concern of the new Chairman who had strong suspicions that my election had been engineered by his opponents. He invited me to dine with him on a floating restaurant on the Thames and this I did. We got to know each other at that meeting and came to realise that far from being opponents we had many ideas in common and that my academic and specialist background complemented his general practice and dental political background.

We agreed to work together to get the Association back on its feet. So began a great friendship which endured for the rest of his life for I admired, liked and respected him. We continued to disagree about the Secretary whose probationary period was coming to an end. Ronnie was impressed with him, whilst I thought that he was a disaster. Both of us expressed our views to Council who, in a majority vote, agreed to recommend to the Representative Board that he be confirmed in office. I asked for my dissent to be recorded in the minutes and so gave notice that I would oppose the recommendation at the Board. At the time I was a member of the Joint Consultants Committee and was surprised when at a meeting of it a President of one of the Royal Colleges, a fellow member of the Committee, began to question me about Alistair Mackie and I learned, in strictest confidence, that he was a candidate for the post of Secretary of the Health Education Council (HEC). I telephoned Ronnie that evening telling him what I had been told whilst not by whom. He interviewed the Secretary and immediately before the Board meeting told me that I had been misinformed. At the meeting which followed we both expressed our opinions on the matter and in the vote which followed the Secretary was confirmed in office.

A few weeks later Ronnie telephoned me to tell me that he was resigning as Chairman of Council as the Secretary had submitted his resignation on being appointed Secretary of the HEC. I was appalled at the news and asked him to do nothing until we had discussed the situation. At dinner the next evening I pointed out my lack of political experience, only just over a year in higher office, and managed to

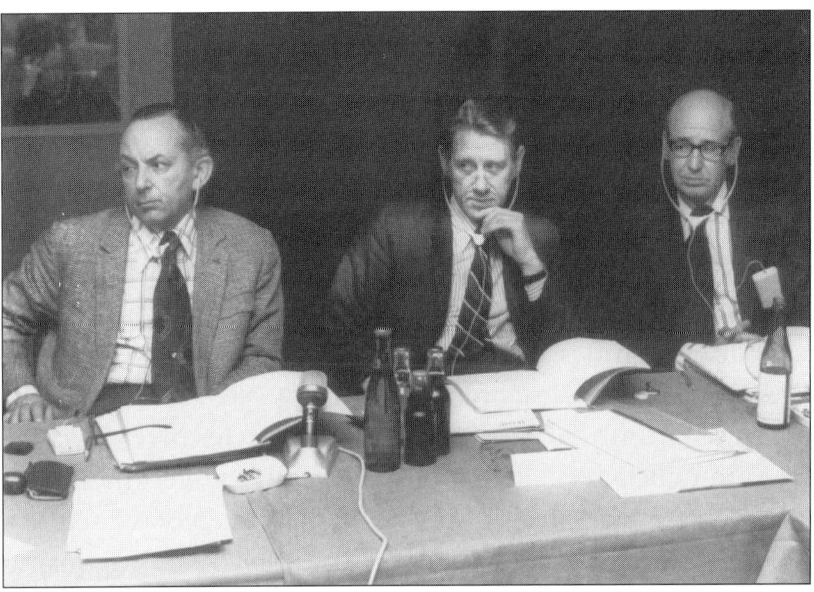

*The UK delegation to the European Regional Organisation of the Federation Dentaire Internationale in 1975. Ronnie Allen is on my left and Gerry Wootliff on my right.*

persuade him to stay on in office in the interests of both the Association and the profession. He tried to persuade me to chair the Selection Committee to appoint a new Secretary but I declined as the terms of reference did not exclude non dentally qualified candidates and I was now convinced more than ever that we could attract a professional colleague of calibre if the terms of service and salary were appropriate. Fortunately the Council agreed to revise both and the post was advertised publicly. It was with mixed feelings that I learned from Ronnie that he had decided to apply for it and had consequently resigned his elected office. His application was successful and I found myself as Chairman negotiating the fine print of his contract with him and his legal advisors. Thus the Association had lost a first class Chairman of

Council but gained an excellent, indeed outstanding, Secretary who adorned the office for the next decade or so. I was also blessed by the election of Gerry Wootliff to serve as Vice Chairman for not only was he on the same wavelength as Ronnie and I but he was very experienced in dental politics and both astute and able in financial matters which I am not. Together the three of us, supported by a regenerated Council, were privileged to lead the Association through very difficult times and one of the most successful periods in its history.

It was a time of political upheaval in the NHS and we were in constant dialogue with successive governments on all aspects of the Health Service. Unfortunately we seldom held the initiative and spent most of our time opposing changes that we considered to be detrimental to the service. Our negotiators were respected in the DHSS for their commitment to the NHS, for doing their homework and their reasoned arguments. For my part I spent many hours in the DHSS HQ at the Elephant & Castle and in the Houses of Parliament. In the company of representatives of the British Medical Association and Ronnie I participated in negotiations with the then Prime Minister, Harold Wilson, once in the Palace of Westminster and the other, an all night session, in No 10 Downing Street. I am afraid that I was singularly unimpressed with him for in my eyes he was an insincere poseur who did not have the best interests of the NHS at heart.

Of all the Secretaries of State I met at such meetings I would rate Barbara Castle the most able and impressive. Although we often differed on various matters I found her to be always immaculately groomed regardless of the hour, an attentive good listener who could be influenced by a reasoned case and invariably courteous. Despite our inevitable differences I liked her very much and always felt that she respected both Ronnie and me. The same could not be said of Sir Keith Joseph who in my humble opinion was the worst holder of that important office that we ever had to deal with. I found him arrogant, aloof and opinionated. He had an annoying habit of winding and unwinding string around a pencil whilst only half listening to what was being said.

On several occasions it was obvious that he was not familiar with the briefs prepared for him by his Civil Service Officers and was ill informed on a number of important matters. One such case was the so called Re-organisation of the NHS which he introduced. Despite much evidence to the contrary being presented by those with practical experience of running and working in the NHS he implemented the management theories of certain non health workers in Brunel University with disastrous results on the Service. Many of those who had submitted carefully researched and exhaustive evidence to him, including the BDA, found our worst predictions coming true but it was about two years before he had the grace to admit it and take remedial action.

During my five year stint as Chairman of Council our main task was keeping the provision of dental care as part of the NHS. In this we succeeded albeit not 'free at moment of use'. Our efforts to get an 'out of hours' Dental Emergency Service were rebuffed by the Government side on grounds of cost. We successfully resisted attempts to exclude dentistry from the terms of reference of the Royal Commission on the NHS to which Professor (now Sir) Paul Bramley, the BDA nominee, was appointed. Many days and weeks were spent by many BDA Committee members and officers preparing, presenting, and submitting evidence to the Royal Commission. The BDA was also one of the bodies which persuaded the Nuffield Foundation to set up a Commission on Dental Education. By the time this was done I was Dean of Dental Studies in Hong Kong where the Dental Project was known to be a major growing point in dental education so much so that the Commission was kind enough to invite me and my colleagues to submit evidence, including our new dental curriculum, and appear before it.

Another major event during my period of office was Britain's accession to the European Common Market, as it was then known. Anticipating this and its implications for the dental profession in the UK, we undertook in-depth studies of both the structure and detailed workings of the EEC and accepted observer status on the EEC Dental Liaison Committee prior to Britain's accession. We became full members as soon as the UK joined and one year later I was elected the President of the Dental Liaison Committee and Ronnie Allen was elected to the office of Secretary General. The task of the Committee was to do the necessary groundwork and draft dental directives to facilitate the freedom of movement and right of establishment of dentists as laid down in the Treaty of Rome. To this end we undertook detailed studies of the very different educational practices, standards and training in all member countries together with the legislation governing the practice of dentistry in each member state. This was a formidable undertaking but the multinational Dental Liaison Committee was rich in talent, ability and knowledge and fully committed to both the EU and its particular task. Every

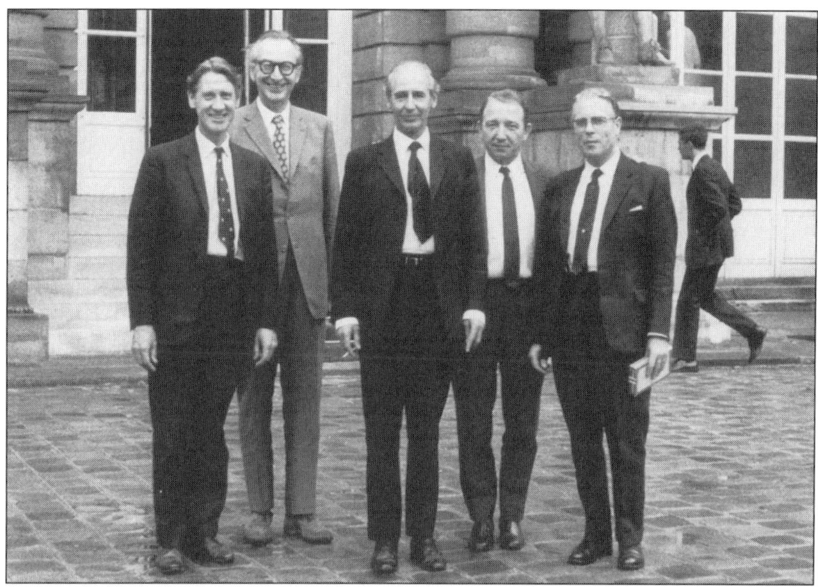

*Representatives of the French and British Dental Associations outside the Palace of Luxembourg in Paris. The French President Dr Jean Jardine is between Ronnie Allen and myself whilst Dr Jacques Charon, their Secretary, is on the right of the then Secretary of the BDA, Jack Peacock.*

delegate was as industrious as they were friendly and the work proceeded apace.

Despite the enormous amount of time, energy and travel involved both Ronnie and I thoroughly enjoyed the experience and agreed to hold office for an unprecedented third year when asked to do so by the Committee. Associated activities included setting up the Association for Dental Education in Europe and explaining both the structure and nature of the EU and relevant developments as they occurred to the dental profession in the UK. Altogether a most enjoyable, worthwhile and satisfying experience which was crowned when Ronnie and I received the congratulations and thanks of our British colleagues, many of whom wondered what our next challenge would be. Ronnie was one of the few close friends who knew at the time that I had decided to resign all my many offices in the UK and go to Hong Kong. Whilst he queried the wisdom of my decision and regretted that we would no longer be working together he understood the reasons for it and wished me well.

Chapter Twelve

# Other Interests and Pursuits

On re-reading what I have written it is immediately apparent to me that I may have given the impression that I was totally absorbed by my professional career to the complete exclusion of all other interests. Nothing can be further from the truth. I freely admit that I am a workaholic and have always tried to give 100% whatever the job in hand but I have thoroughly enjoyed many other interests and pursuits. I was fortunate enough to stumble into the right job for me, academic surgery, and not only did I always look forward to going to work but I missed it terribly when I retired – all three times!

Surgery, though a splendid vocation is an extremely hard mistress. Circumstances outside his control often dictate that the surgeon must make vital clinical decisions without knowing all the relevant facts. An awesome responsibility for being human, he must recognise that his judgement is not always sound and he must live with the consequences. Perhaps the worst aspect of the job is the 'on call' commitment which involves not only one's life but that of family and friends. This is particularly so when a consultant is single-handed, i.e. when he has only junior staff in his speciality who rightly expect him to be available and there for them at times of crisis or difficulty. Thus he lives at the end of a telephone, within a limited radius of his hospital liable to be called out of any family or social occasion at which he must severely restrict any intake of alcohol.

Amid these constraints a good family life and quiet pursuits are essential to happiness. In this I was indeed fortunate for although our homes were very humble whilst I was studying and holding training posts, Heather was a splendid homemaker and ensured that we were always comfortable. She was also an imaginative cook who could quickly conjure up a sustaining and tasty meal despite the rigours of rationing which lasted until the early 1950s. Fortunately I much prefer simple dishes like shepherd's and/or cottage pie to fancy ones. My mouth still drools at the thought of her Cornish pasties, grilled herrings and/or mackerel and her bread and butter puddings! We both shared a love of reading, ballet, music, opera and walking. She was an excellent seamstress who even made shirts for me and a splendid knitter. For my part I was taught to repair my own clothes, darn my own socks and embroider from an early age and still find pleasure in such pursuits. Throughout our lives we both particularly enjoyed student activities and the company of young people. Until she had problems with her back Heather was an excellent lawn tennis player and a Civil Service champion at one time. For my part I enjoyed playing soccer despite being more enthusiastic than skilled. Although I won colours at both my dental and medical schools I failed trials for both United Hospitals and the University. Being rather on the light side I sustained a number of minor injuries until I gave up active participation to become a supporter in my early thirties. In the past I supported Tottenham Hotspur and Newcastle United and for over two decades have endured the anguish of supporting Crystal Palace, though not with the total commitment of both Heather and Tim.

I have always loved the sea and sailing. Heather and I were members of the Little Ship Club and attended meetings and classes there. We also crewed regularly for members who owned boats once crossing the North Sea, in a gale, to spend a month on the Dutch Canals. I helped crew a brick barge in the Thames Barge Race, when we failed to finish, and have been stranded on almost every sandbank in the Colne and Blackwater Estuaries at one time or another. When I was at the Eastman a group of registrars used to charter a boat between us and sail around the Brittany coast and the Channel Islands with Professor Wilkinson as the skipper. We continued this practice for a number of years after leaving that hospital. In Hong Kong I joined the Royal Hong Kong Yacht Club, surely one of the finest and best housed yacht clubs on earth. After obtaining my Master's and Engineer's certificates I bought a third share in a Pandora, called *Pasisana*, and took up yacht racing for the first time with moderate success. Heather and I also had a fifth share in a motorised junk, the *Lady Phyllis*, in which we spent many happy hours.

In the early days of our marriage we used to save for a decent holiday each year and enjoyed sailing as passengers in cargo ships to such destinations as Oslo and the Fiords, Copenhagen, French and Spanish Morocco and up the Seine. When Heather's back problems were too bad for her to sail we took out a second mortgage and purchased a small bungalow in West Town in Hayling Island. It was fun doing it up, it was in a poor state when we got it, and we enjoyed many happy days there. When I retired from Hong Kong we joined a stage purchase scheme and bought a small beach side villa on the outskirts of a small fishing village in the Costa del Sol. After enduring all the usual trials and tribulations of such ventures it has matured into a peaceful haven in the sunshine in which both Tim and Heather found great happiness in their last days. The facilities in the village of Sabinillas have been transformed and as I now live as the spirit moves me and play life by ear I spend a total of almost half a year there.

I also enjoy life in the clubs of my choice. I joined the Savage Club whilst working at the Royal and greatly enjoy its bohemian atmosphere and the company of gifted performers, musicians, writers, artists and sculptors and the like. It must be the most friendly and informal club in London and is most certainly the liveliest. Whilst in Hong Kong I belonged to the United Services Club and the Hong Kong Club in addition to the Yacht Club. Heather and I loved eating in the open air and the poolside lunchtimes spent eating samosas and Ghurka curries in the USC were memorable occasions. The cuisine and facilities of the Hong Kong Club must be second to none and we both enjoyed them to the full and especially so when returning the great hospitality of our Chinese friends. Hong Kong is a gourmet's paradise and Heather was in her element there whether dining in the Peninsula Hotel or an illegal curry house in Kowloon. Soon after returning from Hong Kong I was invited to share the platform with my namesake, the then Foreign Secretary, to discuss the negotiations for the handover of the Colony at the Gents Club, a dining club of catholic membership, at a meeting held in the Traveller's Club. He is a delightful person, whom I had known for many years since his brother was a medical student with me, and a lively informal discussion followed which was enjoyed by all present. I joined the club soon after the meeting and still continue to enjoy my evenings there.

The Territorial Army has also been an important part of my life since I joined it in 1950 whilst a medical student. The 17th (London) General Hospital RAMC (TA) was based at the Duke of York's HQ in Chelsea and had all the special characteristics of a truly volunteer unit. I thoroughly enjoyed the training, especially the Field Training, and the company of all ranks many of whom became lifelong friends, some of whom I describe below. As a unit we worked hard and played hard, often in very isolated places, difficult conditions and awful weather and I must confess that I revelled in it. A number of my fellow officers held senior positions in London Teaching Hospitals and were kind enough to give me individual coaching during my medical studies. Every third year the two week annual camp was held on the Continent and so one saw something of BAOR. When I was appointed in Newcastle I stayed on the establishment of the 17th and trained with them whenever I could, always managing to attend annual camp. For the rest of my training I was attached to 1st (Northern) General Hospital RAMC (TA) based at Fenham Barracks. They were another splendid unit and I was soon made to feel very much at home with them.

Just about the time I returned to work in London the TA merged with the Army Emergency Reserve to form the TA Volunteer Reserve and officers were invited to increase their commitment to the service. The 17th was amalgamated with units in the City of London and Brighton, which became detachments of the main unit which was based at Braganza Street TA Centre in Kennington and renamed 217th (London) General Hospital RAMC (V). This was my Unit

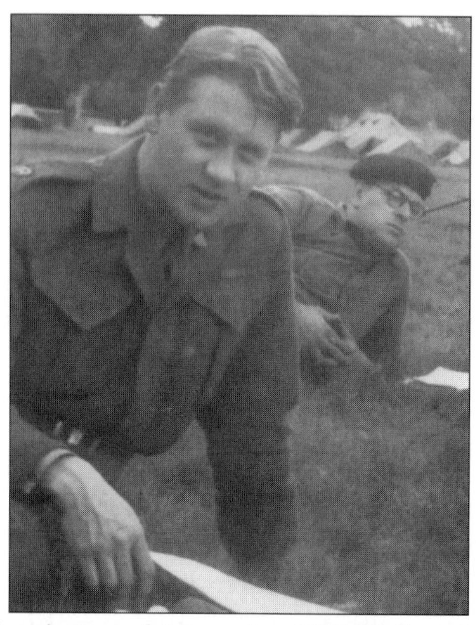

*Briefing during a field exercise. CQMS (later Major) Derek Samuel lies on the grass behind me.*

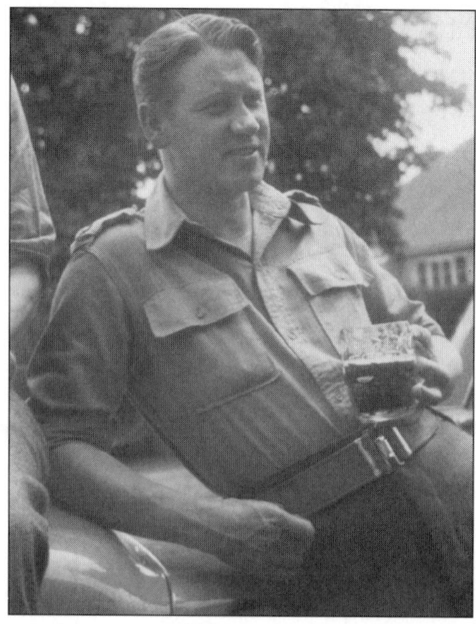

*Relaxing during an off duty period at Annual Camp.*

for the rest of my service and I thoroughly enjoyed being part of it. As an individual I attended a number of courses held at Regular Army establishments in everything from Nuclear Warfare to Messing. I held all manner of jobs in the Unit including being Messing Officer for three years, until a specialist ACC officer was recruited, and President of the Mess Committee for a similar period. The unit had the doubtful privilege of being the General Hospital whose war location was the most advanced one in NATO and we were told that according to the battle plan we were likely to be housing 2000 casualties when overrun by the Russians on the third day of hostilities. Being certain that our potential enemies had read the battle plan and so knew what awaited them down the road we were confident that they would be wise enough to choose another route and comforted ourselves with this thought.

Perhaps the main difference between the Regular and Territorial Armies is that personnel are not posted in or out of their unit in the latter. This means that volunteers serve together for many years and become both friends and team members. As a result morale in TAVR Units is almost universally high. Furthermore in Medical Units, as distinct from Tooth Arm Units, TAVR Commanding Officers are promoted from amongst the TAVR officers serving in the Unit. Tooth arm units are usually commanded by a Regular Officer. Thus as the years went by I served under a succession of COs each of whom held command for three years and was respected and liked by all ranks. As oral and maxillofacial surgery was a Royal Army Dental Corps speciality I was commissioned in that Corps and was not required to re-badge into the Royal Army Medical Corps when I qualified in medicine. In the TAVR at that time there were two Lieutenant Colonel posts in the RADC and after holding one of these for three years dental officers left the active TAVR and were transferred to the Reserve. Seniority was the main factor governing this particular promotion and I became eligible for it long before I wished to cease playing an active role in 217th (London) General Hospital. Thus, with the support and encouragement of successive COs I was allowed to refuse promotion and continue serving in the rank of major. I did this for some time until the Medical Services were unified more closely and under the new policy I became eligible to serve as second in command even though an RADC officer, if selected, after doing my three year stint as a Lieutenant Colonel. So when my turn to be promoted came up again I accepted it, much to the relief of my senior regular colleagues to whom I had been an embarrassment.

During this tour I was selected to attend the RAMC Senior Officers Course at Mychett being the first RADC (TAVR) officer to do so. I thoroughly enjoyed the course and having the advantage over my RAMC (TAVR) colleagues of being senior to them in service and having done a variety of jobs in my unit I did very well on it. As a result I was selected to succeed the second in command of the 217th when he was promoted to command the Unit. Tony Glenister was greatly admired by all and it was my privilege to serve as his 2ic. In civilian life he was a Professor of Anatomy and a renowned embryologist, he was also Dean of Charing Cross Hospital Medical School. When he finished his tour as CO of the 217th he was appointed Advisor on TAVR matters to the Director of Medical Services in the rank of Brigadier General. He later became Master of the Worshipful Society of Apothecaries of which

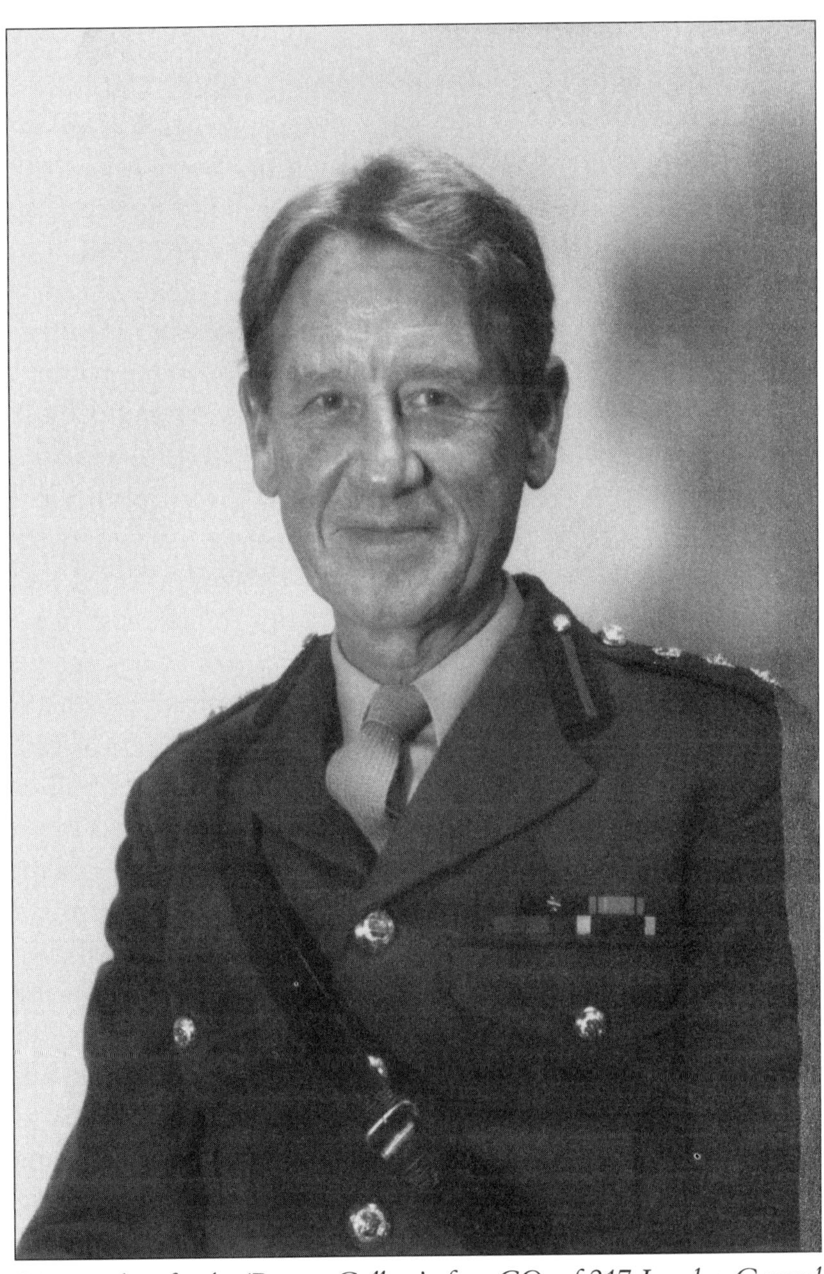

*Picture taken for the 'Rogues Gallery' of ex-COs of 217 London General Hospital (V).*

we were both liverymen. His appointment as CO coincided with an intense drive to streamline and bring up to date the administration of NATO medical units and together we set about this formidable exercise at Unit level. As a result of the efforts of all ranks 217th was awarded the Hospitals Cup being judged the most efficient TAVR General Hospital of the year.

When an officer is promoted to full Colonel he exchanges the collar dogs of his regiment or corps for gorget patches, the colour of which is determined by the branch of the service in which he had previously served. This caused problems when I was selected to succeed Tony as CO as I could not honestly claim to wear the cherry red patches which denote an officer as being 'late RAMC' when I had never served in that Corps. So, as a matter of principle, for I am very proud of my Corps, I said that I would not accept command if I was required to sail under false colours instead of wearing the emerald green denoting that I was 'late RADC'. This did not go down well at all at RAMC HQ at Millbank and I was summoned to discuss the matter with the then Director of Medical Services Lieutenant General Sir Norman Talbot. We discussed the situation and then had lunch together in the RAMC HQ Mess at Millbank during which he told me that his speciality had caused problems for him when he was selected to be DMS. He was an obstetrician and gynaecologist, the busiest medical speciality in the peacetime army! Consequently he was sympathetic to my position and said that he would consult both Queens Regulations and the Regulations of the Medical Services of the Army to see if there was any bar to my wearing green. If there wasn't he would support my application to do so always provided that if there was I would agree to accept

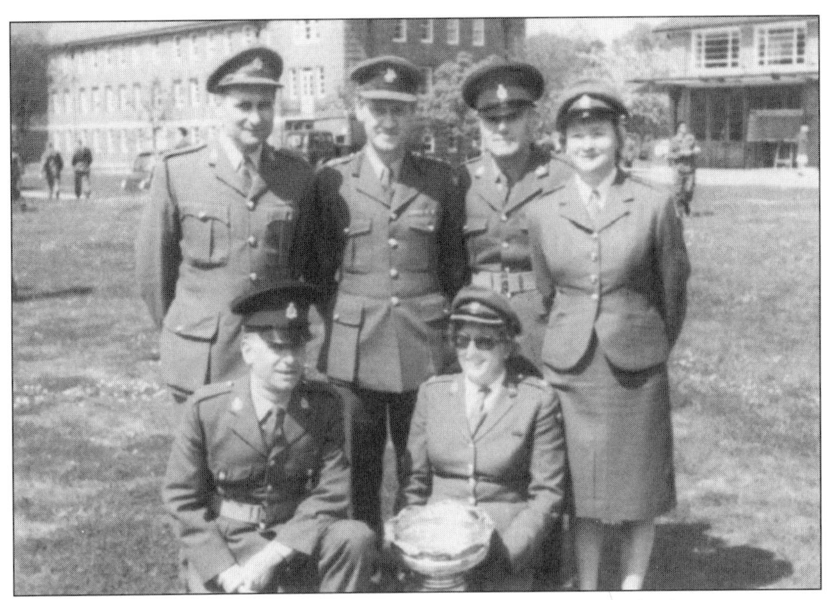

*217 LGH detail after receiving the TA Hospitals Cup.*

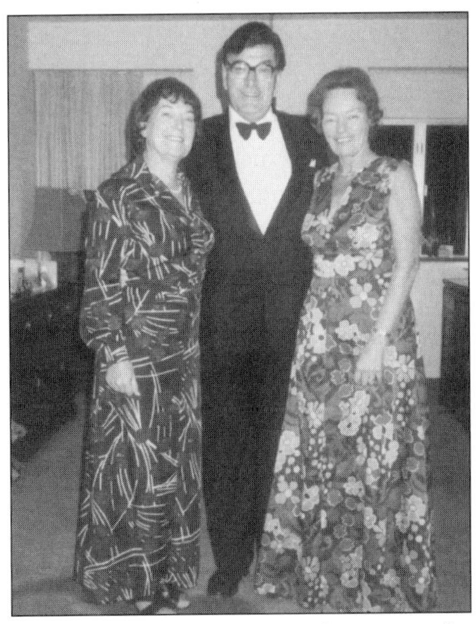

*Derek and Margaret Samuel with Heather in our flat just prior to attending a Christmas dinner in the midst of the ICAC investigation.*

command and wear cherry red. As I had already done the necessary homework I readily accepted his decision. In the event I was allowed to wear green to the dismay of many senior RAMC officers and the delight of my own Corps.

My three years in command were both busy and satisfying as I continued the process of preparing 217th for its war role. The Unit won the Hospitals Cup twice more and was the first TAVR General Hospital to convert an Army School in Germany into an emergency hospital in a couple of days in a PUE (packed until emergency) exercise. I retired from command in October 1975 and served as the first Honorary Colonel Commandant of the RADC and a Colonel on the Regular Army Reserve of Officers (Class 2) until the 30 August 1989. The TA/TAVR is a remarkable and complex volunteer organisation composed of individual units of many kinds, some large some small but each with its own distinctive character. I was privileged to be an active member of it for twenty-five years during which I learned much about life outside the confines of my everyday experiences, participated in activities and events in many places often in adverse weather conditions and forged friendships some of which have lasted for over half a century. Could one ask for more?

My closest friend in the Unit, my 'mukkah' in army parlance, was Derek Samuel. A fine figure of a man he joined the 1st London General Hospital (TA) in 1939 as soon as he was old enough to do so. A few months later the Unit was mobilised and, with all the other volunteers, he was whisked off to war as a Nursing Orderly and was posted to an Indian Army General Hospital commanded by the then Colonel Alex Drummond who went on to become Lieutenant General Sir Alex Drummond and a legendary

DMS. It really is a small world for he was a friend of Professor Wilkinson and crewed alongside me on some of the sailing trips, mentioned earlier, many years later.

Having earned promotion Derek landed in North Africa with the 1st Army in which he served in a Field Ambulance. He saw action in the desert, Sicily and from one end of Italy to the other. Despite his vehicle being blown up several times, usually by land mines, he was lucky enough to survive, having sustained only minor injuries and severe bruising in addition to permanent damage to his hearing. Like many others he was haunted by his wartime experiences to the extent that even in his late seventies he would weep openly when events such as the Festival of Remembrance reminded him of the host of young soldiers that he had been called upon to bury.

After being demobilised he worked as a Charge Nurse in St Stephen's Hospital, Fulham Road and then changed direction and ran a surgical appliance business for the rest of his life. Both he and his lovely Irish wife, Margaret, who is a State Registered Nurse were always there for the Howe family when Heather was unwell, whilst Derek's appliances did much to make life bearable for her when either her neck or her back or both were, as she was wont to say, 'giving her gyp'. The four of us soon became inseparable and we spent at least twenty-five winter villa holidays together in the Algarve, Malta and Corfu. During some of these Heather was far from being well but somehow we always managed to have an enjoyable time in one way or another. Derek was quite definitely a 'one off' serving as he did in the RAMC for over forty years and ending his military career as a Major Quartermaster holding both the MBE and the TD (Territorial Decoration). His distinctive voice and impressive physique ensured that he was soon noted everywhere he went, regardless of the occasion or company that he was in, and he soon became an institution in his Corps of which he was intensely proud.

The irrepressible Peter Lloyd is a highly qualified caterer by trade and is addicted to golf. He always remembers the many jokes that he hears, either whilst raising divots or in the 19th hole. Once he joined the Officers Mess it was fun to be in it regardless of the surrounding conditions. His 'mukkah', another rascal, was the Unit Dental Officer 'Van', Van den Burgh, a Guy's graduate of South African origin who had been a rugby player of some distinction and still bears the trademark stigmata to prove it. Both of them are inveterate practical jokers who are not averse to playing jokes on each other as well as on others. To be in their company is always a tonic and a delight.

Another likeable rogue is Reg Adams who joined the 17th on the same evening that I did, he as a driver in the Royal Army Service Corps, and me as a Captain in the RADC. We met, chatted as we waited on that first evening, and forged a friendship which lasted for a quarter of a century until our paths parted when I retired as CO of 217th. By that time he had rebadged RAMC and attained the rank of Sergeant. A cheerful Cockney he was a shop steward at Briggs Motor Bodies at a time when repeated wildcat strikes there halted the production lines at Ford factories in Dagenham time and time again. He had a remarkable aptitude for being behind lorries at the time when chips of strawberries, tomatoes, mushrooms and the like fell off the back of them and landed, to his great surprise, right in his lap. Remarkably such items often found their way to the Unit and it was his habit to present me with one such item on training nights

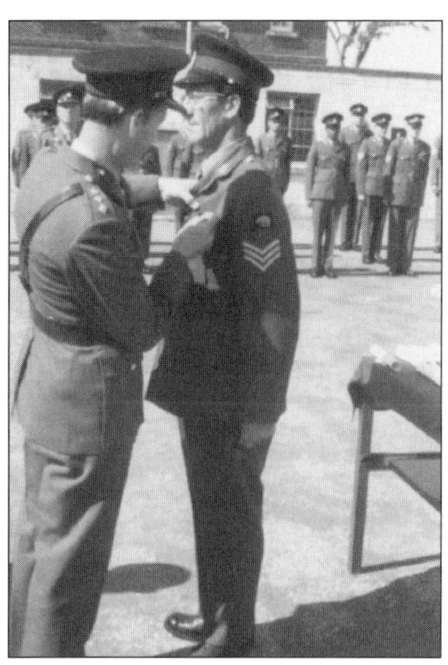

*Investing Sgt Reg Adams with his long service medal.*

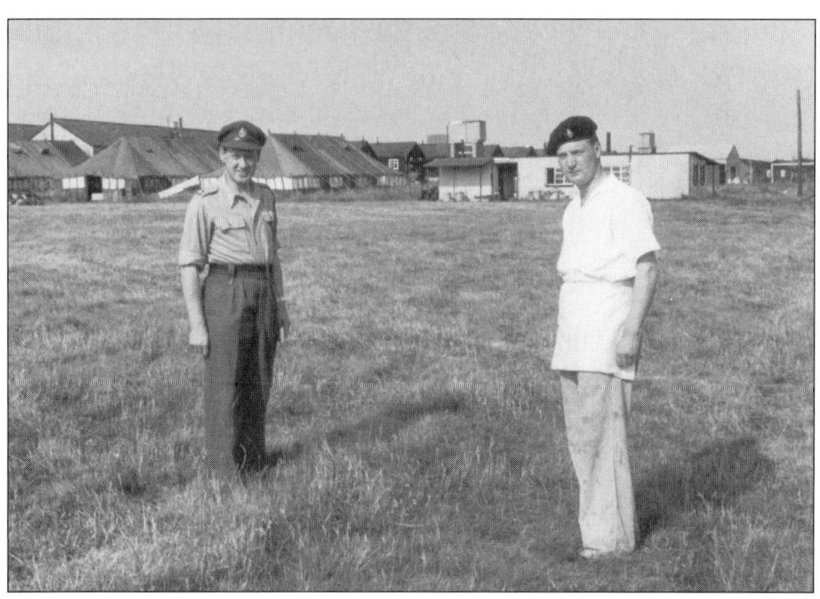

*The Messing Officer and Sgt Cook in front of the cookhouse at camp in Cornwall.*

and to instruct me to take it home as a present for Heather whom he adored and constantly referred to as 'My Ever'!

Whenever we were cold, wet, tired and miserable during field training in a battle area he could be relied upon to appear from nowhere, bearing tea in one hand and barbequed chicken in the other, always explaining that these misguided birds had insisted on committing suicide under the wheels of his Land Rover. For some inexplicable reason there always seemed to be a regular supply of poultry with suicidal tendencies regardless of which battle area or which country we happened to be in. However, when lamb came on the menu I felt it necessary to tell him that I had my doubts that many such four legged creatures had suicidal tendencies or a predilection for his vehicle alone. Only then did he become more discreet about his expeditions to barter with local farmers. I am quite sure that the practice continues as he is an inveterate wheeler dealer!

The morale in TA units is very dependent on the standards of catering within them. Whilst serving as Unit Messing Officer I became very attached to the cooks, an ever cheerful if rather motley collection of scoundrels, none of whom was a cook in civilian life. Indeed there was one dustman and one totter (rag and bone man) amongst them. Despite their complete lack of professionalism they were absolute masters of field cooking and all ranks in the unit lived well. When Peter Lloyd joined the unit and took over the responsibility for messing from me the cooks asked me to continue my custom of going out 'on the town' with them, in civilian clothes, on one night during each fourteen day Annual Camp. This I continued to do and enjoy. The last such occasion was on the very last night before I handed over command of 217th to John Heber. This time they had organised a splendid surprise farewell party for me in the Corporals Mess at which a very good time was had by all but none more than I. Such experiences and friendships confirmed my view that if one has to serve it is better to do so as a unit member rather than as an 'odd bod'.

## Chapter Thirteen

# Epilogue

I FEEL SURE THAT those of my readers who have stayed the course this far will realise why I consider myself to be a very fortunate fellow. From an inauspicious start in humble circumstances I have been lucky enough to have had a full and active life in good company. I had no master plan but listened to the advice of others wiser and worldlier than I, worked hard and accepted challenges and seized opportunities when they presented. I lived at the right time, for though I cannot commend a childhood in the Depression and lost most of my classmates in the 1939-1945 war, I was privileged to be around when the NHS was founded, when the dental profession was transformed from a trade into a profession and when my speciality grew from small beginnings into the valued and respected vocation it is today.

Before the war Rupert Sutton Taylor, a Royal graduate and a Consultant at the Westminster Hospital, was the only dental specialist in the UK to limit his practice, both hospital and private, to Oral Surgery. Most oral surgical procedures were performed by practitioners who undertook other forms of dental treatment in order to make a living. In the absence of antibiotics severe infections of dental origin were rife and could be life threatening and with few exceptions the management of these was the greatest challenge that such colleagues faced. Many confined themselves to performing difficult tooth extractions including the removal of impacted teeth, and the excision of cysts and benign tumours. The setting up of units to deal with war wounds such as gunshot injuries and fractured jaws in both the Armed Forces and the Emergency Medical Service was accompanied by a rapid expansion in both the number of dentists practicing as Oral Surgeons and the range of procedures undertaken by them often in co-operation with Plastic Surgeons. It was into this exciting arena that I was projected as a student house surgeon.

The advent of the NHS provided opportunities for dentists to limit their practice to Oral Surgery as they coped with the aftermath of war and participated in the development of Accident and Emergency Services on a national basis. As one's surgical expertise developed one tried to apply it to the treatment of many other problems. In my case these included the rehabilitation of 'denture cripples', participating as a member of a multidisciplinary team in developing more aggressive operations combined with immediate repair to salvage patients with head and neck cancer previously thought to be incurable and the treatment of facial deformity (Orthognathic Surgery). These and other developments led to the speciality being renamed as Oral and Maxillofacial Surgery.

I was fortunate enough to have parents who, despite all adversity, lived decent lives, had strong social consciences and taught me that education was the road out of poverty despite all the hard work involved and there being no guarantee of success. My primary and grammar school teachers, though firm disciplinarians and hard taskmasters and task mistresses, laid the foundations on which the teachers in my dental and medical schools were able to build. I regard the army as being a university of life in which

I learned much of value from both people and events of many kinds. I certainly grew up whilst serving in it! My experience in general practice taught me that I was ill suited to it and unhappy in it and so I undertook postgraduate training and was fortunate enough to obtain a series of first class training posts under the supervision of outstanding clinicians who taught by example and were masters of their respective crafts. I shall always be indebted to each and every one of them, not least for their taking an interest in me and my future and their wise counsel.

It was purely coincidental that the first advertisement for a Chair in my speciality appeared when I was just about eligible to apply for it. My professional training up to the time I entered University life had been almost entirely governed by the Royal Colleges who were and still are responsible for the maintenance of specialist standards in the NHS. Thus I was clinically rather than academically trained when I became a University employee for the first time and soon found that I had entered a new world in which the criteria for success were as different as were the challenges. I regard myself as having been very privileged to work amongst young people for almost all of my career and to have given them a helping hand in their careers in which in many cases they have been or are eminently successful. Their successes more than compensate one for the pecuniary losses involved in choosing an academic career rather than engaging in private practice. My ex students and ex trainees come from many races and many lands and each of them helped me to become an internationalist. It has been my good fortune to teach, demonstrate or examine in a large number of countries situated in every continent except Antarctica, from which there have been no calls for my services to date.

Life as a dental academic has many facets some of which are not immediately obvious but all of which offer different challenges. I have always believed that one cannot be a good clinical teacher unless one is a good clinician and have rejected the thesis that 'those who can do, those who can't teach'. In the belief that one can only retain and develop clinical skills by constant practice I made this aspect of the job the mainstay of my teaching role. I loved operating and even spent five hours in the operating theatre on my last day in Jordan at the age of seventy-two years and what is more, I thoroughly enjoyed it. I also enjoyed writing three textbooks even though they were merely 'toddlers guides', that is, basic textbooks specifically designed to introduce undergraduate students to a subject, mere teaching tools. I made about fifty other contributions to the scientific literature which varied from case reports and research findings to chapters in textbooks some of which I feel helped advance knowledge. I enjoyed even more teaching my juniors how to make such contributions to knowledge and monitoring their progress by editing their efforts. My personal research was always of a clinical nature for I lack either the flair or the inclination to conduct basic, laboratory or animal research.

After the war the dental schools in the UK were in dire need of upgrading and refurbishment and in common with others I spent many hours playing a role in this process. Unfortunately the Thatcher government halted this progress and indeed pursued a misguided policy of closing both medical and dental schools in the UK thus creating the manpower problems which plague the NHS today. In such a climate I was fortunate enough to play a key role in the establishment of not one but two new dental schools albeit abroad. The contrast between the two Dental Projects could hardly have been more marked. In Hong Kong the government wanted a school of international standard in a very short time and were willing and able to pay for it. They got what they asked for and I tried to ensure that everything was 'state of the art', the curriculum was imaginative and integrated and staffing levels were generous by means of careful planning and staged implementation. In complete contrast when I arrived in Jordan I found that students were already completing the first year of a non existent course for which there was neither a curriculum nor clinical facilities and only a handful of largely inexperienced dental academic staff. Jordan was impoverished, swamped with refugees and trying manfully to cope with problems on every front from road construction and water supply and conservation of scarce resources to education and health services. One could not but admire the way in which this small developing country and its inhabitants were helping themselves and I certainly felt privileged to be given the opportunity to try to assist them overcome at least a few of the problems that confronted them. In the event the Dental Faculty of JUST did produce dental graduates of international quality in about the same time span as did Hong Kong. Many of them undertook postgraduate studies in both the UK and the USA and invariably did well in both their courses and examinations. In the latter their conspicuous success was the subject of much favourable comment from distinguished colleagues in both countries. They now form the core of the teaching staff in JUST, a testament to the wisdom of the policy of localisation and the desire to succeed of both the Jordanians and the Palestinians.

For my part it was both a salutary experience and an educational one. I fought hard to get everything, including computerisation and the use of an electronic microscope in the PPDH for at the time I genuinely believed that such facilities were required to produce top class dental graduates in today's world. My Arabic students proved to me that such a belief was erroneous and that the interface between teacher and student is the essential factor in clinical disciplines for they were just as good graduates as those in Hong Kong who were excellent. The many difficulties and deficiencies that had to be overcome brought staff and students together so much that the 'role model' form of teaching predominated. This, of course, was the way in which I and my fellow students had been educated before University educational practices increased the scientific and research emphasis in both dental and medical education at the expense of the development of clinical skills and compassion for and empathy with patients. There is a tendency today to think that because either a technical procedure is possible or an operation can be performed they are indicated in every case. They are not and treatment should always be fitted to patients and not patients to treatment for they are the most important players in the provision of health care.

Not only was I fortunate enough to find a vocation so interesting, varied and absorbing that I looked forward to going to work every day and did so whether I was being paid or not, but I found a wife who supported me through thick and thin throughout half a century. Although she had to cope with both physical difficulties and depressive illness from the time that she had Tim, she was a woman of great strength and courage who minimised her own problems and went to great pains to hide them from others with conspicuous success. She also looked after Tim superbly in the last two or three years before his untimely death in

August 1997 at the age of thirty-nine, a tragic loss from which she never really recovered before she passed away some four months later, having urged me repeatedly to write this account of my life before I joined her. I am happy to say that she was right, as usual, for I have found it to be a cathartic experience which has helped me greatly and made me realise what a lucky fellow I have been, I commend the practice to others. Having, at one time or another been a Fellow of nine or ten educational bodies or learned societies I feel entitled to call myself a Fortunate Fellow hence the title of this, my swansong.